Bladder Cancer

CANCER SURVEYS

Advances and Prospects in Clinical, Epidemiological and Laboratory Oncology

SERIES EDITOR: J Tooze
Consulting Editor: L M Franks
Editorial Assistant: C E Sinclair

Associate Editors

W Bodmer	A Harris	J Ponten
V Beral	NR Lemoine	B Stillman
H Calvert	P Nurse	N Wright
C Dickson	MJ Owen	J Wyke
	T Pawson	

Published for the

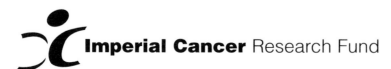

Imperial Cancer Research Fund

Bladder Cancer

Guest Editors
R T D Oliver
M J Coptcoat

COLD SPRING HARBOR LABORATORY PRESS 1998

CANCER SURVEYS
Bladder Cancer
Volume 31

Cover and book design by Leon Bolognese & Associates, Inc.

All Cold Spring Harbor Laboratory Press publications may be ordered directly from Cold Spring Harbor Laboratory Press, 10 Skyline Drive, Plainview, New York 11803-9729. Phone: Continental US & Canada 1-800-843-4388; all other locations (516) 349-1930. FAX: (516) 349-1946. All other locations: (516) 349-1930. FAX: (516) 349-1946. E-mail: cshpress@cshl.org. For a complete catalog of all Cold Spring Harbor Laboratory Press publications, visit our World Wide Web Site http://www.cshl.org/

Contents

Introduction: Clonal Evolution in Bladder Cancer: A Scientific and Clinical Perspective   1
R T D Oliver and M J Coptcoat

Risk Factors in Clonal Development from Superficial to Invasive Bladder Cancer   5
Jaime Landman and Michael J Droller

Squamous Change in Bladder Cancer and Its Relevance to Understanding Clonal Evolution in Development of Bladder Cancer   17
S Baithun, P Daruwala and R T D Oliver

Malignancy Associated Papillomaviruses and Morphology of Human Bladder Cancer   29
R T D Oliver, J Breuer, A M E Nouri and S Campo

Molecular Genetics of Bladder Cancer: Pathways of Development and Progression   49
Margaret A Knowles

Molecular Biological Changes in Bladder Cancer   77
Khaver N Qureshi, John Lunec and David E Neal

Clinical Evaluation of Immunotherapy: Are There Differences between Papillary and Flat In Situ Bladder Cancer?   99
Donald L Lamm

Clonal Development of Bladder Cancer and Its Relevance to the Clinical Potential of HLA Antigen and *TP53* Based Gene Therapy   109
A M E Nouri, R T D Oliver and V H Nargund

The Role of Surgery in the Multimodality Treatment of Bladder Cancer   129
Malcolm J Coptcoat and R T D Oliver

Radiotherapy and Chemotherapy for Invasive Bladder Cancer   149
Miland Javle and Derek Raghavan

Future Directions   161
Malcolm J Coptcoat and R T D Oliver

BIOGRAPHICAL NOTES   165
INDEX   167

Introduction: Clonal Evolution in Bladder Cancer: A Scientific and Clinical Perspective

R T D OLIVER[1] • M J COPTCOAT[2]

[1]Department of Oncology, QMW School of Medicine & Dentistry, St Bartholomew's Hospital, West Smithfield, London EC1A 7BE; [2]Department of Urology, King's College Hospital, Denmark Hill, London SE5 9RS

Today, progress in genetics and cytogenetics is making it clear that most cancers develop by a form of Darwinian like somatic evolution so that there is preferential survival of the most malignant clone, with increasing anaplasia and metastases being associated with the accumulation of genetic damage. There is clear evidence that this is in part influenced by inheritance of genes that cause deficiency of DNA repair or immune response. Environmental exposures that cause DNA damaging and/or immunosuppressive effects provide the other principal dimension of causation. This cumulative damage leads to cancer principally by causing non-function of DNA replication suppressor genes and overexpression of mutated cellular proliferation oncogenes in association with increasing expression of oncofetal antigens marking a reversion of cell to infantile phenotype. Bladder cancer has contributed much to this modern viewpoint of cancer development because it is one of the first cancers, after cancer of the scrotum, to be associated with an industrial chemical exposure, one of the first cancers where genetic inheritance has been shown to have a specific genetic mechanism that increases risk of cancer (ie the fast acetylator phenotype) and the first human tumour cell type in which transfectable human oncogenes were demonstrated, as well as the first tumour type where a greater than 50% 10 year "cure" of early stage cancer has been demonstrable from the use of immunotherapy. Today, with bladder cancer increasing, particularly in the superficial preinvasive stages due to increased access to simplified diagnosis with flexible cystoscopy, without any evidence of a reduction in mortality, this volume of *Cancer Surveys* aims to re-examine bladder cancer from both a scientific and a clinical perspective in an attempt to set a new agenda for the next millennium.

Though long regarded as a model for public health intervention and screening based on the successful interventions in the dye and rubber industries, bladder cancer as it presents today rarely shows evidence of an obvious aetiological risk factor apart from smoking. Droller, in his clinical perspective overview of bladder cancer epidemiology, will focus specifically on this issue and the evidence on how far epidemiological risk factors have been associated with the clonal extremes of bladder cancer—that is, the superficial and invasive variants.

Pathologically, most bladder tumours are transitional cell carcinomas. There is, however, increasing recognition of the prognostic importance associated with the metaplastic variants showing squamous and glandular differentiation as part of the evidence for clonal evolution in this disease. Baithune and colleagues review the importance of these morphological variants and in particular the contribution of bilharzia in the development of the pure squamous subtype that has such an economic importance in Africa. The significance of finding that squamous change in bovine papillomavirus induced bladder tumours is a surrogate indicator of papillomavirus replication provides an indication of why squamous change may be important in human bladder cancer. Long before cystoscopy confirmed it in vivo, pathologists were well aware that the majority of bladder cancers had a papillary morphological phenotype. It is 60 years this year since the classical experiments of Shope in wild and inbred rabbits first demonstrated that under most circumstances papillomavirus behave as benign stimulators of cellular proliferation whose cell cycle is tightly coupled with the differentiation process of the epithelial cell, mostly in the skin. More recently it has become apparent that they are also able to induce tumours in some animals by affecting bowel, bladder, oral and genital epithelia. In Shope's original studies it was well established that the more malignant life threatening phenotypes were only expressed when there was repeated exposure to a carcinogen or the genetic background facilitated malignant progression. With the increasing understanding of papillomavirus biology, particularly from studies of bovine papillomavirus, Breuer and colleagues' review of human and bovine papillomavirus studies in bladder cancer will focus on the extent to which such viruses could be causative factors in the variable morphology of bladder tumours and on their potential for use as vaccines.

Since the first transfection studies led to the identification of the *RAS* oncogene, the complexity of interacting mechanisms that regulate cell proliferation has increased markedly. After colon cancer, bladder cancer is the most widely studied cancer for cytogenetic evidence to support the concept of clonal evolution. Knowles, in her chapter, updates this area, particularly the relevance of the data on 9q losses that seem to separate the papillary and flat/solid cancers early in tumour development. In addition, her chapter discusses the potential that knowledge about the molecular mechanisms involved in tumour progression offers for development of new approaches to treatment.

This theme is further developed by Neal and colleagues who focus on the increasing understanding of the importance of growth factors, angiogenesis and metalloproteinases in early stepwise clonal initiation of all tumour types and the considerable potential for therapeutic interventions that this has opened up.

With 10 year follow-up studies now published providing the first irrefutable evidence that immunological manipulation can improve survival in early stage cancer, it is clear that superficial bladder cancer offers a significant opportunity as a test bed of new approaches to immunotherapy. Lamm, in his chapter, reviews the data that establish the superiority of bacille Calmette-Guérin over chemotherapy in both the papillary and flat tumour subtypes and focuses on some of the early attempts to develop less toxic approaches.

There has long been evidence from animal models that gene therapy could play a significant part in cancer, though progress in applying it to human cancer has been slow, in part because of medicolegal issues and in part because of the complexity of the genetic damage that modern cytogenetics has revealed. Oliver and Nouri review these issues and develop a rationale as to how gene therapy could be investigated in bladder cancer.

The importance of a thorough grounding in surgical science in order to appreciate the best way of maximizing the benefits of surgery, which is still the best single method in cancer treatment, is often underemphasized. With new evidence from molecular biology demonstrating the effects of tissue repair cytokines on tumour growth and prolonged anaesthesia on immune response and new polymerase chain reaction techniques to detect tumour cell dissemination in the blood stream and lymph nodes, increasing attention is being paid to minimal surgical intervention and the benefits of endoscopic approaches to surgery. Coptcoat, in his chapter, reviews these developments as well as the creativity of surgeons in evolving new approaches to reconstructing the bladder that are doing much to improve quality of life following treatment.

Although not renowned as the most chemosensitive tumour in humans, with palliative responses to combination treatment in more than 70% of patients and durable, complete remissions in more than 5% of patients, bladder cancer is certainly as sensitive as breast and ovarian cancer to conventional dose treatment in patients with terminal metastatic disease. Despite this, chemotherapy has as yet no established role in early invasive cancer. With the increasing complexity of molecular targets for the newer generation of chemotherapeutic drugs, a new era for combination therapy is opening up and the chapter by Javle and Raghaven focuses on these developments. As well as reviewing past experience, this chapter looks to the future potential of these drugs and their interaction with radiation, which, it has to be remembered, remains the best single method of non-surgical therapy against primary invasive tumours.

Risk Factors in Clonal Development from Superficial to Invasive Bladder Cancer

JAIME LANDMAN • MICHAEL J DROLLER

Department of Urology, Mount Sinai School of Medicine, New York

Introduction
Cigarette smoking
Occupational exposures
Other factors
Summary

INTRODUCTION

Bladder cancer is the sixth most common neoplasm world wide, affecting approximately three times as many males as females (Wingo *et al*, 1995). Each year in the USA approximately 54 000 new cases of bladder cancer are diagnosed, and over 12 000 deaths are attributed to bladder cancer (Parker *et al*, 1997). In men, bladder cancer is the fourth most common cancer, accounting for 10% of all new cancer cases. In women, bladder cancer is the eighth most common malignancy and accounts for 4% of all cancers. The lifetime risk of developing bladder cancer has been estimated to be 2.8% for white men, 0.9% for black men, 1% for white women and 0.6% for black women.

These gender and racial differences suggest either a distinct genetic susceptibility to bladder cancer or differences in environmental exposures between men and women and between races. Schairer *et al* compared 3000 cases identified through the Surveillance, Epidemiology and End Results registries to community control subjects. After adjustment for smoking and high risk occupation, the risk of developing transitional cell carcinoma among whites was 1.6 times that of blacks (Schairer *et al*, 1988). In contrast, Silverman and colleagues examined risks for bladder cancer associated with occupation among white and non-white men and concluded that the overall risk was similar in the two groups (Silverman *et al*, 1989b).

In 1895 Rehn reported three cases of bladder cancer in workers in the aniline dye industry (Rehn, 1895). This has been taken as the first documented association between bladder cancer and exposure to environmental carcinogens. Although familial cases of bladder cancer have been reported (Fraumeni and Thoman, 1967), most evidence has implicated exogenous factors in the development of carcinoma of the bladder. These have included cigarette smoking, as the most consistently and strongly associated with the development of

Cancer Surveys Volume 31: *Bladder Cancer*
© 1998 Imperial Cancer Research Fund. 0-87969-529-3/98. $5.00 + .00

bladder cancer, occupational exposures to chemicals such as aromatic amines, and infections.

The prognosis of an individual with bladder cancer varies substantially according to the grade and stage of the tumour at diagnosis. An estimated 70% of bladder cancers when diagnosed involve only the mucosa (T_a). The 5 year survival rate for individuals presenting with this form of bladder cancer is over 80%. In contrast, tumours that have penetrated the lamina propria (T_1) have been associated with a 50–78% 10 year survival for grade II and III lesions, respectively (Fitzpatrick, 1989). Grade I is rarely seen in tumours that are not confined to the mucosa. As tumours progress to higher stages, which are associated with muscle invasion (T_2 and T_3), 5 year survival falls to below 50%.

There is substantial evidence for the existence of two separate types of bladder cancer. For example mucosally confined papillary tumours only rarely progress to invasive disease, despite the high frequency of recurrence (Heney *et al*, 1983). In contrast, some forms of mucosally confined cancer (carcinoma-in-situ) may become progressive and occasionally even metastasize without ever assuming a superficial papillary appearance (Herr, 1989). This suggests that carcinoma-in-situ represents a biologically different diathesis than papillary, mucosally confined, bladder cancer (Jones and Droller, 1993). Furthermore, some cancers, even though muscle infiltrative, respond to conservative bladder preserving treatments (Hudson and Kramer, 1981) and do not appear as potentially aggressive as some that have penetrated the bladder wall only as deeply as the lamina propria. This suggests that the initiation of carcinogenesis may lead to the development of processes that are proliferative but produce cells that are unlikely to progress, or processes that are proliferative but produce cells that also have the ability to penetrate the bladder wall and ultimately to metastasize. Although these distinct diatheses may represent a continuum in the expression of malignant transformation from the lesser to the more aggressive forms, they could also represent distinct pathways of carcinogenesis.

It has been suggested that epidemiological risk factors known to be associated with the development of bladder cancer may be differentially associated with these different forms of bladder cancer. Host factors may also have a role in the distinctive forms of cancer. We have reviewed the literature regarding the epidemiology of bladder cancer with respect to distinctions that may be correlated with the development of indolent versus aggressive disease. Although this topic has had only limited study, there appears to be some evidence suggesting associations between cigarette smoking, occupational exposure, host factors and the different types of bladder cancer that occur.

CIGARETTE SMOKING

Cigarette smoking has been strongly associated with the development of bladder cancer in more than 30 case-control studies. The relative risk varies from 2 to 10 depending on the amount of cigarette use. Cessation of cigarette smoking has been suggested to lead to an estimated 30–60% reduction in bladder cancer risk during the first 2–4 years (Hartge *et al*, 1987). Smoking unfiltered cigarettes increases the risk by 50%, the filter presumably limiting exposure to some of the carcinogens contained within cigarette smoke.

Although the majority of cigarettes smoked around the world are composed of blond (bright or flue cured) tobacco, black (burley or air cured) tobacco is still much used in the Mediterranean countries of Europe and in Latin America. Five case-control studies in Italy, France, Argentina and Uruguay have reported the relative risk of transitional cell carcinoma to be two to three times higher for smokers of black tobacco than for smokers of blond tobacco (Iscovich *et al*, 1987; Vineis *et al*, 1988; Clavel *et al*, 1989; Silverman *et al*, 1989; De Stefani *et al*, 1993).

Black tobacco smoke contains higher concentrations of aromatic amines and has been associated with greater urinary mutagenicity than blond tobacco (Mohtashamipur *et al*, 1987; Patrianakos and Hoffman, 1979). Paolo *et al* demonstrated a beneficial effect of smoking cessation in smokers of both black and blond tobacco, with a 50% decline in risk of developing bladder cancer over the first three years (Vineis *et al*, 1988). Men who discontinued the use of blond tobacco ultimately had no significant increase in risk over that in non-smokers. In contrast, although cessation of smoking reduced overall risk of bladder cancer in smokers of black tobacco, they still ultimately remained more than twice as likely as non-smokers to develop bladder cancer. However, the rapid initial decrease in risk associated with cessation of smoking of either form of tobacco is consistent with a late stage of action in the progression of carcinogenesis.

The continued elevation of risk for bladder cancer in smokers of black tobacco also suggests that the bladder epithelium in this population may have undergone additional alteration and that an elevated risk for development of bladder cancer was maintained. Whether this implies a relationship between invasive bladder carcinoma and type of tobacco smoked has yet to be evaluated.

The mechanism by which cigarette smoking produces bladder cancer has not been defined. It is probably related to the numerous chemicals in cigarette smoke, such as polycyclic aromatic hydrocarbons, aromatic amines and unsaturated aldehydes, which have been associated with the genesis of bladder cancer in other settings (Clayson and Cooper, 1970; Price, 1971). For example there is considerable evidence that aromatic amines, especially 4-aminobiphenyl and *o*-toluidine, may underlie the association between cigarette smoking and bladder cancer (Silverman *et al*, 1989a). Other aromatic amines may also be present as part of the pyrolysis products that occur.

Such primary aromatic amines occur in smoke at nanogramme levels per cigarette. However, patterns of metabolism and macromolecular binding in exposed subjects and animal models suggest that aromatic amines require metabolic activation by complex, often competing, pathways before they exert a DNA binding effect and carcinogenicity (Miller and Miller, 1981). The formation of metabolic intermediates in the liver through N-hydroxylation is catalysed in humans predominantly by cytochrome P450IA2 (Butler *et al*, 1989). This enzyme activity shows an apparently trimodal distribution in different populations and has prompted the tentative designation of slow, intermediate and rapid P450IA2 (N-hydroxylation) phenotypes (Butler *et al*, 1992). Although there is still no proof that the N-oxidation phenotype is due to genetic polymorphism, it is possible that certain individuals may activate aromatic amines to their carcinogenic states more readily. This population could therefore be more susceptible to the deleterious effects of cigarette smoke.

Thus, the metabolites of arylamines may enter the circulation, react covalently with haemoglobin in erythrocytes and become disseminated throughout the body, where they may ultimately react with urothelial DNA. The latter would be the critical event in the initiation of bladder carcinogenesis. Other studies of aromatic amine induced bladder cancer have demonstrated higher levels of these haemoglobin adducts in patients described as slow acetylators (Vineis, 1990). N-acetyltransferase is an enzyme involved in the deactivation of some arylamines, the urinary excretion of which is increased after acetylation. Human populations show a characteristic genetically based polymorphism for the activity of this enzyme, with about 50% of subjects being "slow" acetylators and 50% "fast" acetylators. Cartwright *et al* published a case-control study of 111 bladder cancer cases and 207 controls (one group of healthy subjects and one group of urological patients) (Cartwright *et al*, 1982). They demonstrated that slow acetylators were significantly more likely to develop bladder cancer than fast acetylators. Overall, there appears to be a 30–50% increase in the proportion of slow acetylators among bladder cancer patients. Additionally, it has been demonstrated that the concentration of haemoglobin adducts in slow acetylators is significantly higher than in rapid acetylators (Bartsch *et al*, 1990).

Elucidation of an association between either superficial or invasive bladder cancers and cigarette smoking has recently become a point of interest. Hayes *et al* evaluated the relative risk for the development of both invasive and superficial bladder cancers as a result of smoking (Hayes *et al*, 1993). An increased risk for both superficial and invasive bladder cancer without a clear cut distinction between them was confirmed. Although the relative risk for bladder cancer appeared to be marginally greater for superficial than for invasive disease, the dose response pattern was more distinct for invasive bladder cancers. When patients aged under 60 were considered alone, the relative risk for the development of invasive bladder cancer with cigarette smoking was greater than that for superficial cancer.

There have been no attempts to explain why only smokers under 60 are more susceptible to the development of invasive transitional cell carcinomas. In a review by Jones and Droller (1993), a putative schema for the evolution from superficial to invasive bladder cancers involved a progression of multiple genetic alterations at sites on chromosomes 9 and 17. Superficial (T_a) tumours were frequently associated with losses or deletion of chromosome 9, whereas other defects were observed in higher grade, higher stage tumours (Olumi *et al*, 1990). This evidence suggests that initial inactivation of genes on chromosome

9 may be an early event whereby the absence of tumour suppressor genes permits the production of a proliferative tumour diathesis. This may be followed by multiple sequential inactivations of other genes on separate chromosomes, which may lead to an invasive and possibly metastatic phenotype. The earlier exposure of the population aged under 60 may increase the probability of the occurrence of multiple "hits" that may be needed for the development of the invasive phenotype.

Sturgeon and colleagues evaluated the relative risk for the development of bladder cancer as a result of smoking and stratified their results by grade (Sturgeon *et al*, 1993). They demonstrated a clear dose dependent increased risk with cigarette smoking, increasing exposure being associated with increased grade of disease (Table 1). Additionally, increased doses of cigarette smoke resulted in increased risk for the development of high stage tumours. The highest relative risk from cigarette smoking was for development of extravesicular disease, followed closely by an increased relative risk for tumours invading the musculature. The smallest increase in relative risk was found for superficial tumours. Specifically, the relative risks for tumours extending beyond the bladder, tumours invading the musculature and superficial tumours for smokers of more than 40 cigarettes per day were 6.8, 4.3 and 3.0, respectively.

Sturgeon suggested several explanations for these observations (Sturgeon *et al*, 1994). One suggestion is that cigarette smokers may be less likely than non-smokers to obtain medical care, which could interfere with early cancer detection. Thus, differential use of medical services by smoking status could explain why smokers may be proportionally more likely than non-smokers to be diagnosed with invasive bladder cancer if it is assumed that the cancer had a greater

TABLE 1. Smoking and bladder cancer stage (Sturgeon *et al*, 1994)

	Relative risk			
	Non-invasive (pT$_a$) n=1045	**Submucosal (pT$_1$) n=258**	**Muscle invasive (pT$_{2/3}$) n=191**	**Extension beyond bladder (pT$_4$) n=89**
Never smoked	1.0	1.0	1.0	1.0
Ex smoker				
<20/day	1.5	1.5	1.3	2.9
≥20/day	1.6	2.8	2.0	3.8
Current smoker				
<20/day	1.6	2.7	3.0	3.6
20–39/day	2.8	3.1	3.7	6.1
≥40/day	3.0	5.5	4.3	6.8

chance to progress since it remained undetected for longer. However, if the concept of different pathways of cancer development and their corresponding likelihood of progression is valid, this would not support this suggestion. In contrast, the data also suggest a role for certain compounds in cigarette smoke to act at a late stage in bladder cancer progression. This suggests that smoking may cause late chromosomal damage, which helps to promote the transition from superficial disease to more aggressive forms of bladder cancer capable of invasion. This "crossover" effect in producing a different pathway is more consistent with the concept of multiple but interrelated pathways of bladder cancer development and progression. Another explanation is that superficial and invasive bladder cancers are distinct entities, with the latter being more closely associated with cigarette smoking. These different possibilities have yet to be fully explored.

Another report evaluating smokers demonstrated an association between cigarette smoking and three factors relating to the severity of bladder cancer—tumour stage, grade and number of recurrences (Thompson *et al*, 1987). They demonstrated a significant association between smoking and all variables. Within this military population 79% of the patients found to have bladder cancer demonstrated a smoking history. Cigarette smokers were found to have significantly more aggressive disease, with almost one third of patients manifesting muscle invasive bladder cancer. Only 14% of non-smoking patients were found to have invasive disease. Non-smoking patients also demonstrated lower grade and fewer recurrences than patients with a history of cigarette smoking.

Cigarette smoking represents the most significant preventable cause of bladder cancer in the US population. Approximately 15 000 cases of bladder cancer could be eliminated and approximately 5000 lives saved each year when calculations based upon risk are considered (Wynder and Goldsmith, 1977; Silverberg, 1985).

OCCUPATIONAL EXPOSURES

Stimulated by Rehn's work on the link between occupational exposure and bladder cancer, similar reports appeared in Switzerland and England in the early 1900s. Hueper *et al*, in 1938, demonstrated that the industrial chemical 2-naphthylamine could induce bladder cancer in dogs that was identical to lesions seen in humans (Hueper, 1938). Studies in British workers in the 1950s by Case *et al* identified a 30 times increased risk of bladder cancer in individuals exposed to arylamines (Case *et al*, 1954). A long latency period was identified between initial exposure and subsequent development of bladder malignancy. Although exceptions have been noted, bladder cancer typically manifests 15–40 years after the initial exposure to chemicals in the occupational setting.

Most bladder carcinogens are aromatic amines. The most investigated compounds are 2-naphthylamine, benzidine and 4-aminobiphenyl. Other carcinogenic chemicals are derived from aromatic amines. These include azo dyes derived from benzidine, which were first shown to induce bladder cancer in kimono painters in Japan who licked their brushes to obtain fine points (Yoshida *et al*, 1971).

Although many work environments have been studied for an increased risk of bladder cancer, strong evidence of increased associations exists for very few occupations. These include dye workers, aromatic amine manufacturing workers, leather workers, rubber workers, painters, truck drivers and aluminum workers (Silverman *et al*, 1992).

The proportion of bladder cancer in men caused by occupational exposures has been estimated at 18–35% (Matanoski and Elliot, 1981). Using an estimate of 25% from a National Cancer Institute study (Silverman *et al*, 1989a) and projections from bladder cancer incidence and mortality (Wingo *et al*, 1995), it can be estimated that nearly 25% of cases (over 12 000) and 25% of deaths (2500) annually are a result of occupationally caused bladder cancer.

Few studies have evaluated the relationship between the types of bladder cancer that occur and the particular type of occupational exposure and specific increases in tumour stage. In a case-control study the relative risk associated with aromatic amine bladder carcinogens was found to be virtually identical for superficial and invasive disease (1.7 and 1.5, respectively) when all men were considered (Hayes *et al*, 1993). The occupation associated risk was found to be elevated in younger men but not in men aged 75 or more years. In the population of men studied who were younger than 60, however, the relative risk for invasive tumours was almost three times higher than the relative risk for superficial disease.

Sturgeon and colleagues evaluated patients in high risk occupations including painters, motor vehicle drivers, railroad workers, hairdressers and barbers, petroleum processing workers, rubber processing workers, stationary engineers and firemen, blasters, powdermen and writers (Sturgeon *et al*, 1994). They demonstrated an increased relative risk for both superficial and invasive bladder cancer but no differences between different stages. Additionally, when patients were stratified by age no consistent pattern was discerned. However, the risk for muscle invasive and metastatic bladder cancer was higher in the non-white population than in the white population. This observation may be explained by differential access or use of health care services by race, with delay in obtaining medical attention by the non-white population. Risk of disease invading muscle and beyond was also slightly elevated among those with less than a high school education.

In 1978 attention was drawn to bladder cancer in West Yorkshire, UK, by high mortality figures published by the Office of Population Censuses and Surveys. These studies indicated that the bladder cancer mortality for males and females of industrialized Huddersfield County was extremely high for people of working age for the period of 1969 to 1973, whereas the corresponding figures for nearby Bradford County were significantly lower. The main carcinogens in Huddersfield were found to be naphthylamine, magenta, auramine and benzidine (Glashan *et al*, 1981). Evaluation of these populations by two separate groups yielded interesting differences between the presentation and extent of tumour (Cartwright *et al*, 1980; Glashan *et al*, 1981). Bladder cancers in Huddersfield had significantly poorer prognosis, with 12%, 11% and 15% decreased survival at 1, 2 and 5 years, respectively (Cartwright *et al*, 1980). These survival differences were not explained by age at presentation, since patients presented at slightly younger ages in Huddersfield.

The noted differences in survival were most striking when stratified by stage. Remarkably, survival for stages T_2 to T_4 were similar in exposed and non-exposed patients. However, major survival differences in these series were seen in patients with stage T_1 bladder cancers. Cartwright *et al* (1980) demonstrated four stage T_1 deaths (4%) in Bradford County, while there were nine stage T_1 deaths (20%) in Huddersfield. The slightly younger age range, the occurrence of apparently later stages despite earlier presentation and the poorer prognosis of apparently milder cases in Huddersfield suggested that these bladder cancers may reflect unknown biological differences when contrasted with the bladder cancers of Bradford County.

An exfoliative urine cytology screening programmme was established in Huddersfield County, the results of which have been reviewed (Glashan *et al*, 1981). Patients with abnormal urine cytology were evaluated cystoscopically and systematically followed for prolonged periods. There was a remarkably consistent progression from urothelial dysplasia to carcinoma-in-situ and finally to invasive bladder tumours. Changes seemed to be progressive, with disruption of the basement membrane ultimately yielding invasive tumours. There was no explanation for the unusually high association of occupational exposure and progression of bladder cancers to invasive forms. However, as with cigarette smoking, it is possible that bladder cancers associated with occupational exposures may result from more severe chromosomal damage. These cancers may therefore progress more quickly to invasive phenotypes.

Brooks *et al* evaluated occupational risk of bladder cancer in a large population of workers in Missouri (Brooks *et al*, 1992). High risk employment was defined as employment previously established as having an elevated relative risk by an earlier study in Missouri, or employment which had a relative risk of 1.5 or greater in at least two case-control studies since 1980. After adjustment for both age and smoking high risk employment was associated with advanced tumour grade. However, there did not appear to be a similar association between occupational risk category and stage, since stage was similar for both high risk and control populations. When only workers aged under 60 were considered there was an association between high risk occupation and both high grade and high stage tumours. The risk of high stage cancer with high risk occupation was approximately doubled in younger men.

Despite the limited number of studies evaluating the relationship between occupational exposure and alteration in patterns of presentation and natural history of bladder cancers, there seem to be surprisingly similar conclusions between studies. Occupational exposure increases the risk for bladder cancer such that higher grade and stage cancers are observed. Additionally, there are alterations in the biology of bladder cancers induced as a result of occupational exposure. Finally, bladder cancers in high risk occupations found in men under 60 seem to be of higher stage than those found in the general population.

OTHER FACTORS

Many factors have been linked with increased risk for bladder cancer, including analgesics, coffee and artificial sweeteners. Surprisingly, there have been few attempts to evaluate the risk for alterations in disease presentation or biology as a result of these exposures. One study evaluated 1860 bladder cancer cases and determined that there were no changes in stage of presentation or tumour grade with exposure to coffee or artificial sweeteners (Sturgeon *et al*, 1994). There is increasing evidence that host factors may have an important role in the development of bladder cancer in these instances. However, these factors may not have substantial influence in the development of bladder cancer in the general population. This may affect associations that exist but that consequently are difficult to ascertain.

SUMMARY

Bladder cancer has classically been associated with exogenous risk factors, and a large literature has identified risk factors associated with the genesis of transitional cell carcinoma. Only recently have efforts been made to identify host factors and to evaluate possible changes in tumour presentation and biology, including grade and stage, in association with these risk factors. The available literature appears to demonstrate alterations in tumour biology associated with environmental carcinogens. Various studies have suggested a consistent upgrading of bladder cancer stage and grade as a result of cigarette smoking and high risk occupational exposures. It is important, however, that all factors associated with increased risk for bladder cancer be more extensively evaluated in assessing the validity of this concept.

References

Bartsch H, Caporaso N, Coda M *et al* (1990) Carcinogen hemoglobin adducts, urinary mutagenicity, and metabolic phenotype in active and passive cigarette smokers. *Journal of the National Cancer Institute* **82** 1826–1831

Brooks DR, Geller AC, Chang J and Miller DR (1992) Occupation, smoking, and the risk of high-grade invasive bladder cancer in Missouri. *American Journal of Industrial Medicine* **21** 699–713

Butler MA, Iwasaki M, Guengerich FP and Kadlubar FF (1989) Human cytochrome P450pa (P-450IA2), the phenacetin O-deethylase, is primarily responsible for hepatic 3-demethylation of caffeine and N-oxidation of carcinogenic arylamines. *Proceedings of the National Academy of Sciences of the USA* **86** 7696–7700

Butler MA, Lang NP, Young JF *et al* (1992) Determination of CYP1A2 and acetyltransferase phenotypes in human populations by analysis of caffeine urinary metabolites. *Pharmacogenetics* **2** 116–127

Cartwright, RA, Glashan RW and Gray B (1980) Survival of transitional cell carcinoma cases in two Yorkshire centres. *British Journal of Urology* **52** 497–499

Cartwright RA, Glashan RW, Rogers HJ *et al* (1982) The role of N-acetyltransferase in bladder carcinogenesis: a pharmacogenetic epidemiological approach to bladder cancer. *Lancet* **ii** 842–845

Case RAM, Hosker ME, McDonald DB and Pearson JT (1954) Tumors of the urinary bladder in workmen engaged in the British chemical industry: role of analine, benzidine, alpha-naphthylamine and beta-naphthylamine. *British Journal of Industrial Medicine* **11** 75–104

Clavel J, Cordier S, Baccon-Gibod L and Hemon D (1989) Tobacco and bladder cancer in males: increased risk for inhalers and black tobacco smokers. *International Forum on Cancer* **44** 605–610

Clayson DB and Cooper EH (1970) Cancer of the urinary tract. *Advances in Cancer Research* **13** 271

De Stefani E, Barrios E and Fiero L (1993) Black (air-cured) and blond (flue cured) tobacco and cancer risk III: oesophageal cancer. *European Forum on Cancer* **29A** 801–803

Fitzpatrick JM (1989) Superficial bladder cancer: natural history, evaluation, and management. *AUA Update Series* **8** 82

Fraumeni JF and Thoman LB (1967) Malignant bladder tumors in a man and his three sons. *Journal of the American Medical Association* **201** 507

Glashan RW, Wijesinghe DP and Riley A (1981) The early changes in the development of bladder cancer in patients exposed to known industrial carcinogens. *British Journal of Urology* **53** 571–573

Hartge P, Silverman D, Hoover R *et al* (1987) Changing cigarette habits and bladder cancer risk: a case-control study. *Journal of the National Cancer Institute* **78** 1119–1125

Hayes, RB, Friedell GH, Zahm SH and Cole P (1993) Are the known bladder cancer risk factors associated with more advanced bladder cancer? *Cancer Causes and Control* **4** 157–162

Heney NM, Ahmen S, Flannagan MJ *et al* (1983) Superficial bladder cancer: progression and recurrence. *Journal of Urology* **130** 1083

Herr HW (1989) When is a cystectomy necessary in carcinoma in situ? In: Murphy GP and Khoury S (eds). *Therapeutic Progress in Urologic Cancers*, p511, Mosby Publishing, New York

Heuper WC, Wiley FH and Wolfe HD (1938) Experimental production of bladder tumors in dogs by administration of beta-naphthylamine. *Journal of Industrial Toxicology* **20** 46–84

Hudson HC and Kramer SA (1981) Transitional cell carcinoma of the renal pelvis: rare occurrence in young males. *Urology* **18** 284–286

Iscovich J, Castelleto R and Esteve J (1987) Tobacco smoking, occupational exposure and bladder cancer in Argentina. *International Forum of Cancer* **40** 734–740

Jones PA and Droller MJ (1993) Pathways of development and progression in bladder cancer: new correlations between clinical observations and molecular mechanisms. *Seminars in Urology* **11** 177–192

Matanoski GM and Elliot EA (1981) Bladder cancer epidemiology. *Epidemiology Review* **3** 203–229

Miller EC and Miller AJ (1981) Searching for the ultimate chemical carcinogens and their reactions with cellular macromolecules. *Cancer* **47** 2327–2345

Mohtashamipur E, Norpoth K and Lieder F (1987) Urinary excretion of mutagens in smokers of cigarettes with various tar and nicotine yields, black tobacco, and cigars. *Cancer Letters* **34** 103–112

Olumi AF, Tsai YC, Nichols PW *et al* (1990) Allelic loss of chromosome 17 distinguishes high grade from low grade transitional cell carcinomas of the bladder. *Cancer Research* **50**

7081–7083

Parker SL, Tong T, Balder S and Wingo PA (1997) Cancer statistics 1997. *CA A Cancer Journal for Physicians* **47**: 5–27

Patrianakos C and Hoffman D (1979) Chemical studies of tobacco smoke LXIV: on the analysis of aromatic amines in cigarette smoke. *Journal of the Analysis of Chemicals* **3** 150–154

Price JM (1971) Etiology of bladder cancer, In: Maltry E (ed). *Benign and Malignant Tumors of the Urinary Tract*, pp 189–251, Medical Examination Publishing, New York

Rehn L (1895) Blasengeschwulste bei anilinarbeitern. *Archiven Klinical Chimica* **50** 588–600

Schairer C, Hartge P, Hoover RN *et al* (1988) Radical differences in bladder cancer risk: a case control study. *American Journal of Epidemiology* **127** 1027–1037

Silverberg E (1985) Cancer statistics, 1985. *Cancer* **35** 19

Silverman DT, Levin LI and Hoover RN (1989A) Occupational risks of bladder cancer in the United States: I, white men. *Journal of the National Cancer Institute* **81** 1472–1479

Silverman DT, Levin LI and Hoover RN (1989b) Occupational risks of bladder cancer in the United States: II, nonwhite men. *Journal of the National Cancer Institute* **81** 1480–1483

Silverman DT, Hartge P, Morrison AS and Devessa SS (1992) Epidemiology of bladder cancer. *Hematology Oncology Clinics of North America* **6** 1–30

Sturgeon SR, Hartge P, Silverman DT e*t al* (1994) Associations between bladder cancer risk factors and tumor stage and grade at diagnosis. *Epidemiology* **5** 218–225

Thompson, UN, Peek M and Rodriguez F (1987) The impact of cigarette smoking on stage, grade and number of recurrences of transitional cell carcinoma of the bladder. *Journal of Urology* **137** 401–403

Vineis P, Esteve J, Hartage P, Hoover R, Silverman DT and Terrachini B (1988) Effects of timing and type of tobacco in cigarette-induced bladder cancer. *Cancer Research* **48** 3849–3852

Vineis P, Caporaso N, Tannenbaum SR *et al* (1990) Acetylation phenotype, carcinogen-hemoglobin adducts and cigarette smoking. *Cancer Research* **50** 3002–3004

Wingo WJ, Tong T and Bolden S (1995) Cancer statistics, 1995. *Cancer* **45** 8–30

Wynder EL and Goldsmith R (1977) The epidemiology of bladder cancer: a second look. *Cancer* **40** 1246–1249

Yoshida O, Harada T, Miyagawa M *et al* (1971) Bladder cancer in workers of the dyeing industry. *Igayu No Ayumi* **79** 421–430

The authors are responsible for the accuracy of the references.

Squamous Change in Bladder Cancer and Its Relevance to Understanding Clonal Evolution in Development of Bladder Cancer

S BAITHUN • P DARUWALA[1] • R T D OLIVER

Departments of Histopathology and Medical Oncology, St Bartholomew's and The Royal London Hospitals, London EC1A 7BE

Introduction
Squamous metaplasia in transitional carcinoma
Incidence of squamous metaplasia in human and bovine bladder cancer
    Historical aspects
    Co-factors in bilharzia associated squamous bladder cancer
    Cytology and cytogenetics of bilharzial bladder cancer
Summary

INTRODUCTION

In the west the majority of bladder cancers arise in men over age 65 (Harnden and Parkinson, 1996), and the dominant cell morphologically is the transitional cell (about 80%), with pure squamous cell (5%), adenocarcinoma (1–2%) and sarcomatoid variants (less than 1%) making up most of the remaining cases (Young, 1996). These figures are in striking contrast to those for bladder tumours arising in the areas of the world (predominantly the Middle East and Africa) where there is bilharzial infection of the bladder (Ferguson, 1911). The age at onset in these countries is much earlier (often before age 50). The male:female ratio depends on degree of exposure to bilharzia, being 11.8:1 in Egypt (Makhyoun *et al*, 1971) where the males predominate among workers on the land, and 1.75:1 in Mozambique (Prates and Gillman, 1959) where the women also work on the land. The predominant morphological type associated with bilharzial infection is pure squamous carcinoma, and most tumours arise remotely from the trigone in more than 95% of cases (Khafagy *et al*, 1972), whereas most transitional cell carcinomas (TCCs) arise close to the ureteric orifices or near the trigone (Harnden and Parkinson, 1996).

In recent years, with improvements in light microscopy and the availability of an increasing range of monoclonal antibodies, there has been increasing recog-

[1]Present address: Department of Urology, Western Infirmary, Edinburgh

nition that a substantial minority of TCCs have "metaplastic" components (Starklint *et al*, 1976). The commonest of these is squamous metaplasia, which in one series occurred in more than 50% (Martin *et al*, 1989). The commonest other well recognized variants are those showing trophoblastic elements (Jenkins *et al*, 1990) or neuroendocrine elements (Grignon *et al*, 1992), though occasional cases have areas of multiple morphological variants, as in germ cell cancers, and can express glandular, squamous and even cartilaginous/osteoid "metaplastic" change in the same tumour (Lam, 1995).

Prompted by reports from study of bovine papillomavirus (BPV) associated transitional cell bladder tumours which demonstrate that infectious virus expression occurs only in keratinized squames (Campo, 1997) and that a minority of bladder tumours show human papillomaviruses (HPVs) (Nouri *et al*, this volume), this paper re-examines the issue of squamous metaplasia in transitional cell cancers and compares these findings with the morphology of BPV tumours and reviews the literature on the role of bilharzia in induction of squamous change in bilharzial associated bladder cancer.

SQUAMOUS METAPLASIA IN TRANSITIONAL CARCINOMA

Squamous metaplasia has long been noted to be a concomitant component of a small minority of bladder cancers and associated with a poor prognosis (Hope-Stone *et al*, 1984). With improved fixation and staining it has become apparent that squamous metaplasia is present in a higher proportion than previously appreciated, in one series being demonstrated in 58% of invasive tumours (Jenkins *et al*, 1990). A similar phenomenon has been observed in respect of histopathological staging of Hodgkin's disease, when recognition of previously overlooked finely collagenized avascular fibrous bands led to an increase in the frequency with which nodular sclerosing Hodgkin's disease was diagnosed from 28% to 67% (Chelloul *et al*, 1972). The association of squamous metaplasia with poor prognosis is in part a reflection of the fact that it occurs more frequently in invasive tumours (Table 1), being rarely seen in the non-invasive pT_a tumours (Fig. 1), even when poorly differentiated (Fig. 2). Its presence in invasive tumours (Fig. 3) is predominantly deep within tumour masses and less frequently in the areas of urothelium surrounding the actual tumour in contrast to the findings in the classical squamous cancers associated with bilharzial infec-

TABLE 1. Squamous metaplasia in superficial and early invasive human transitional cell carcinoma of the bladder

	No of cases	% with squamous metaplasia
G_1pT_a	5	20
$G_{2/3}pT_a$	6	33
PT_1	4	75
$\geq pT_2$	2	100

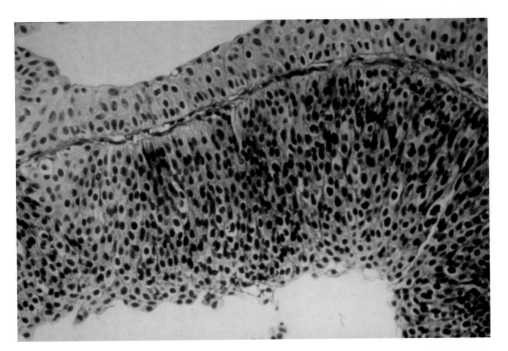

Fig. 1. G_1pT_a bladder transitional cell carcinoma

tion, where it is common to find areas of squamous metaplasia in the neighbouring areas of "normal" urothelium surrounding the tumour (Ishak *et al*, 1967). That the poor prognosis associated with expression of squamous metaplasia is not just due to its association with invasive tumours comes from an analysis of response to radiotherapy in a group of invasive tumours classified on the basis of expression of squamous metaplasia and beta human chorionic gonadotropin (hCG) (Table 2). It is clear, first, that presence of squamous metaplasia is a strong predictor of failure to respond to radiation, since only 24% of positive cases achieved complete remission, compared with 85% of those without squamous metaplasia. The presence of hCG expression in the tumour cells outside the area of squamous metaplasia was seen to be an interactive risk factor for radiation response (Table 2), since only 7% with both factors responded, compared with 34% with squamous metaplasia in the absence of β-hCG expression. With increasing interest in the idea that β-hCG might function as an autocrine growth factor, possibly via interaction with epidermal growth factor receptor, and new information that granulocyte colony stimulating factor may also function as an autocrine growth factor in these tumours (Tables 3, 4), there is clearly more to be learned from study of bladder cancer morphology that might give insights into the derangements of cell replication. Equally important, given the increasing recognition of the importance of a functioning *TP53* gene in determining response to radiation and chemotherapy (Sarkis *et al*, 1995), would be to repeat these studies of squamous metaplasia with screening for *TP53* mutations.

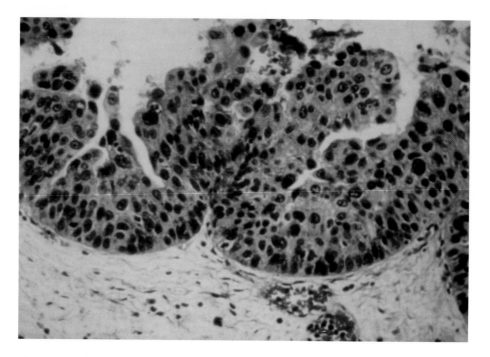

Fig. 2. G_3pT_a bladder transitional cell carcinoma

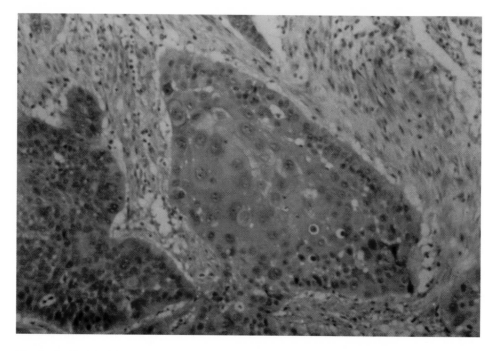

Fig. 3. G_3pT_{2+} bladder transitional cell carcinoma with squamous metaplasia

INCIDENCE OF SQUAMOUS METAPLASIA IN HUMAN AND BOVINE BLADDER CANCER

As discussed by Nouri *et al* (this volume), the association of infectious papillomavirus production with keratinization and development of squamous change in the skin is a major reason for interest in what is behind the high incidence of squamous metaplasia in both transitional and squamous carcinoma. As yet there has been no association of squamous metaplasia with human papillomavirus expression in our own series, although a limited review of samples from the bovine studies by Campo *et al* (1985) has been begun to investigate this further. So far the limited studies have demonstrated that the frequency in bovine tumours is similar to that of invasive human tumours (Table 5), although more work needs to be done to investigate the significance of these changes with virus persistence and the "hit and run" hypothesis (Campo *et al*, 1985).

Historical Aspects

That bilharzial cystitis was associated with squamous bladder cancer was suggested by Ferguson's report on 40 cases (Ferguson, 1911) and confirmed in Egypt (Makhyoun *et al*, 1971), Mozambique (Prates and Gillman, 1959), Zimbabwe (Gelfand, 1950), South Africa (Kisner, 1973), Sudan (Malik *et al*, 1975), Zambia (Bhagwandeen, 1976) and Iraq (Talib, 1970). That bilharzial infection could induce "papillomatous" change in rhesus monkey bladders within 3 months of infection was demonstrated in 1920 (Fairley, 1920), but it was only in 1980 that studies in baboon demonstrated that a synergistic interaction was needed between the bilharzial parasite and carcinogen to produce the malignant phenotype (Hicks *et al*, 1980). The high frequency of bacterial infection associated with nitrosamine induction in areas of endemic bilharzial infection (Laughlin *et al*, 1978) suggests that bacterial infection could be an additional co-factor in the human disease since it has been demonstrated in squamous tumour arising spontaneously in areas of low bilharzial incidence.

The powerful effect of bilharzial infection as a promoting agent for transformation comes from a comparison of age incidence (Makhyoun *et al*, 1971) of bilharzial (males 43, females 41) and non-bilharzial bladder cancer in the same population (males 61, females 58), although what evidence exists suggests that there is a minimum of 10 years from first bilharzial infection to tumour induction (Makar, 1955).

Co-factors in Bilharzial Associated Squamous Bladder Cancer

Bilharzial infection is clearly a most significant promoter of squamous bladder cancer. However, in Zimbabwe non-squamous TCC is more common in white people, because of its association with smoking (Vizcaino *et al*, 1994), than squamous cell carcinoma was in blacks, 70% of whom had bilharzial infection

TABLE 2. Interaction between squamous metaplasia and β-hCG expression as prognostic factor for invasive bladder response to radiotherapy

	β-hCG positive		β-hCG negative	
	No of cases	% CR after radiation	No of cases	% CR after radiation
Squamous metaplasia positive	28	7	44	34
Squamous metaplasia negative	8	75	45	87

CR = Complete response

(Gelfand, 1950). This is an indicator that bilharzial infection is not an absolute guarantee of tumour induction. Moreover, in parts of Africa, such as Nigeria (Attah and Nkposong, 1976) and Uganda (Dodge, 1962), squamous carcinoma can occur at a high frequency in the absence of bilharzial infection. The high frequency of urethral stricture in such cases, often associated with chronic persistent urinary tract infection, suggests that the common factor is the constant inflammatory process, with epithelial cell death and replacement mitosis reducing the time available for DNA repair. A similar process has become accepted as the principal mechanism for the association between *Helicobacter* infection and induction of carcinoma of the stomach (Forman, 1996). In that tumour, however, there is no induction of squamous change as the first step in tumour development. However, since squamous metaplasia is the characteristic precursor lesion for cervical (Eifel *et al*, 1997; Mullokandov *et al*, 1996), oral (Mao *et al*, 1996; Califano *et al*, 1996) and bronchial (Chung *et al*, 1996) cancers, and since in one study 73% of bilharzial associated squamous cancers had evidence of squamous metaplasia in the mucosa adjacent to the tumour and similar change was demonstrable in 28% of TCCs (Ishak *et al*, 1967), there is clearly a need for more study of the genetics of this change in different tumour types. This is particularly so since studies of squamous metaplastic areas in bronchial epithelium from patients with lung cancer have shown selective loss of heterozygosities that are also present in more advanced forms of squamous lung cancer (Chung *et al*, 1995). With the undoubted association of squamous change in more than 85% of cases of cervix cancer associated with HPV infection (Brule *et al*, 1993), with increasing evidence for HPV involvement in 30–50% of squamous oral cancer (Shindoh *et al*, 1995) (Snijders *et al*, 1996), possibly 10–20% of lung cancers (Bejui-Thivolet *et al*, 1990; Yousem *et al*, 1992) and possibly also 10–15% of bladder cancers (Nouri *et al*, this volume) and with no information on HPV infection in bilharzial squamous carcinoma, there are clearly further areas to explore with regard to the development of squamous metaplasia. The observation of a "hit and run" process in BPV tumours (Campo *et al*, 1985) needs to be further investigated in HPV related tumours, particularly given that HPV can be detected in 30% of squamous skin cancer arising in

TABLE 3. Risk factors affecting survival in patients with T$_3$ bladder cancer (Daruwala, unpublished)

Variable	No of cases (total 60)	Survival >2 y (%)	Univariate analysis using group	Univariate analysis as a continous variable
Serum albumin <37 g/L	10	30	p<0.8	0.148
Serum albumin ≥37 g/L	50	52		
Creatinine <120 μmol/L	22	45	p<0.58	0.03
Creatinine <120 μmol/L	35	46		
Anaemia	30	47	p<0.5	0.003
Normal haemoglobin	30	50		
Alkaline phosphatase >115 IU/L	22	27	p<0.2	0.001
Alkaline phosphatase ≤115 IU/L	34	56		
Granulocyte count >7.5 x 10^9	18	17	p<0.001	0.001
Granulocyte count <7.5 x 10^9	42	62		
Lymphocyte count <1.5 x 10^9	23	26	p<0.025	0.003
Lymphocyte count >1.5 x 10^9	37	62		

immunosuppressed individuals but in only 3% of spontaneously arising tumours (Kawashima *et al*, 1990). The ever increasing number of HPV subtypes and evidence that class II histocompatibility linked genes are involved in susceptibility/resistance (Han *et al*, 1992; Davies and Stauss, 1997) suggests that there is clearly more to learn from this area. A single anecdotal report of durable complete response after treatment with synthetic recombinant HPV protein vaccine in cervix cancer is particularly encouraging in this respect (Borysiewicz *et al*, 1996).

Cytology and Cytogenetics of Bilharzial Bladder Cancer

Schistosomiasis remains one of the major public health problems of the tropics, possibly affecting as many as 200 million people. The late presentation of bilharzia associated bladder cancer is a constant problem in all countries with a high incidence of schistosomiasis (Groeneveld *et al*, 1996). A recently developed dot enzyme linked immunosorbent assay (ELISA), using a monoclonal antibody CK1K10 raised against keratinized grade 1 squamous cell carcinoma, is showing promise in the clinic, with a specificity of 90% and clear superiority to cytology (Attallah *et al*, 1996). As previous studies using conventional cytology screening have demonstrated impressive reduction of advanced cases (El-Bolkainy *et al*, 1982), the dot ELISA assay could be very advantageous in the

TABLE 4. Granulocytosis and lymphopenia as interacting risk factors in T_3 bladder cancer (Daruwala, unpublished)

	No of cases	2 y survival (%)
Granulocytes ≥7.5/lymphocytes ≤1.5	10	20
Granulocytes ≥7.5/lymphocytes >1.5	9	34
Granulocytes <7.5/lymphocytes ≤1.5	14	43
Granulocytes <7.5/lymphocytes >1.5	27	81

tropical setting because it is cheap, does not require sophisticated equipment or highly trained staff and can be performed in less than 30 minutes.

It also could have potential in selecting samples for molecular analysis in the field. There is increasing evidence that molecular studies are opening up a new perspective on this disease. These are, however, showing that there are some similarities to TCC, in that fluorescence in situ hybridization with repetitive alpha satellite probes for chromosomes 9 and 17 has suggested that monosomy 9 may be an early chromosomal change in urothelium of the bilharzia infested bladder and a predictor of incipient carcinoma, as in pure TCCs. Further insight into schistosomal bladder cancer epidemiology has come from study of *TP53* mutations. Warren *et al* (1995) compared the proportion of base pair substitutions (BPS) among 34 mutations in schistosomal bladder cancer with literature reports on non-schistosomal bladder cancer. The proportion of BPS at CpG dinucleotides was significantly higher in schistosomal than in non-schistosomal bladder cancer (18/34 vs 25/103, p=0.003). This observation, and the fact that there was a bias away from mutations at exons 7/8 towards exons 5/6, led the authors to suggest that the difference was due to nitric oxide exposure, long suspected to be involved in tumours arising in association with chronic bacterial infection (Laughlin *et al*, 1978; Mirvish, 1995).

SUMMARY

Using conventional morphological assessment, squamous change in bladder epithelium has been observed in 73% of bilharzial associated squamous cancers but only 28% of pure transitional cancers. However, more detailed studies of patients with TCC suggest that the latter figure may be an underestimate, since in one series it was reported to be more than 50%. The most significant risk factor for development of squamous carcinoma in the bladder is chronic persistent bacterial cystitis, although in the areas of the world where bilharzia is endemic this infestation also increases the risk of both squamous bladder cancer and chronic bacterial cystitis. Although it is clear that carcinogens are involved as co-factors in transformation from squamous metaplasia to cancer, the fact that in Zimbabwe one author has observed that TCC is more frequent in whites than squamous cancer is in bilharzia infected blacks is evidence that other unidenti-

TABLE 5. Squamous metaplasia in human and bovine bladder cancer

	Unselected ≥pT$_2$ TCC (n=125)[a]	Tumours from HLA antigen study (n=17)[b]	Bovine BPV induced bladder tumours (n=7)[c]
≥pT$_2$	100%	12%	86%
Squamous metaplasia	58%	47%	57%
Haemangiosarcoma	0%	0%	43%

[a]Jenkins *et al*, 1990
[b]Nouri *et al*, 1997
[c]Campo *et al*, 1985

fied risk factors are involved. This is increasing evidence for involvement of HPV subtypes in cervix, oropharynx and lung cancer. As all three of these tumours are associated with squamous metaplasia, there could be a case for investigation of bladder squamous tumours for HPV involvement. This is particularly so given the observation of the "hit and run" type of transient infection in cattle that develop BPV associated tumours and the tenfold difference (30% vs 3%) in frequency of HPV detection in squamous skin tumours developing in immunosuppressed individuals compared with those arising spontaneously.

With new technology for cytological screening techniques using dot ELISA and evidence of differences in *TP53* mutations that support the involvement of nitrous oxide, it is clear that there is more to learn from study of this tumour type that may be of general interest in understanding the clonal development of cancer.

References

Attah EB and Nkposong EO (1976) Schistosomiasis and carcinoma of the bladder: a critical appraisal of causal relationship. *Tropical Geographical Medicine* **28** 268–272

Attallah AM, el-Didi M, Seif F, el-Mohamady H and Dalbagni G (1996) Comparative study between cytology and dot-ELISA for early detection of bladder cancer. *Amerian Journal of Clinical Pathology* **105** 109–114

Bejui-Thivolet F, Liagre N, Chignol MC, Chardonnet Y and Patricot LM (1990) Detection of human papillomavirus DNA in squamous bronchial metaplasia and squamous cell carcinomas of the lung by in situ hybridization using biotinylated probes in paraffin-embedded specimens. *Human Pathology* **21** 111–116

Bhagwandeen SB (1976) Schistosomiasis and carcinoma of the bladder in Zambia. *South African Medical Journal* **50** 1616–1620

Borysiewicz LW, Fiander A, Nimako M et al (1996) A recombinant vaccinia virus encoding human papillomavirus type-16 and type-18, E6 and E7 proteins as immunotherapy for cervical cancer. *Lancet* **347** 1523–1527

Brule AJC van den, Snijders PJF, Meijer CJLM and Walboomers JMM (1993) PCR-based detection of genital HPV genotypes: an update and future perspectives. *Papillomavirus Reports* **4** 95–99

Califano J, Riet P van der, Westra W *et al* (1996) Genetic progression model for head and neck cancer: implications for field cancerization. *Cancer Research* **56** 2488–2492

Campo MS (1997) Bovine papilloma virus and cancer. *British Veterinary Journal* **154** 175–188

Campo MS, Moar MH, Sartirana ML, Kennedy IM and Jarrett WF (1985) The presence of bovine papillomavirus type 4 DNA is not required for the progression to, or the maintenance of, the malignant state in cancers of the alimentary canal in cattle. *EMBO Journal* **4** 1819–1825

Chelloul N, Burke J, Motteram R, Capon J Le and Rappaport H (eds). *Report of Histological Analysis. Histocompatibility Testing*, pp 769–771, Munksgaard, Copenhagen

Chung GT, Sundaresan V, Haselton P *et al* (1995) Sequential molecular genetic changes in lung cancer development. *Oncogene* **11** 2591–2598

Chung GT, Sundaresan V, Haselton P *et al* (1996) Clonal evolution of lung tumours. *Cancer Research* **56** 1609–1614

Davies DH and Stauss HJ (1997) The significance of human leukocyte antigen associations with cervical cancer. *Papillomavirus Reports* **8** 43–50

Dodge OG (1962) Tumours of the bladder in Ugandan Africans. *International Journal of Cancer* **18** 538–552

Eifel PJ, Berek JS and Thigpen JT (1997) Cancer of the cervix, vagina and vulva, In: Vita VD, Hellman S and Rosenberg S (eds). *Cancer: Principles and Practice of Oncology*, vol 5, pp 1433–1456, Lippincott Raven, Philadelphia, Pennsylvania

El Bolkainy MN, Chu EW, Ghoneim MA and Ibrahim AS (1982) Cytologic detection of bladder cancer in a rural Egyptian population infested with schistosomiasis. *Acta Cytologica* **26** 303

Fairley NH (1920) A comparative study of experimental bilharziasis in monkeys contrasted with the hitherto described lesions in man. *Journal of Pathology and Bacteriology* **23** 289

Ferguson AR (1911) Associated bilharziosis and primary malignant disease of the urinary bladder, with observations on a series of forty cases. *Journal of Pathological Bacteriology* **16** 76–94

Forman D (1996) Helicobacter-pylori and gastric cancer. *Scandinavian Journal of Gastroenterology* **31** 48–51

Gelfand M (1950) *Schistosomiasis in South Central Africa, Cape Town and Johannesburg*, pp 91–99, Juta and Co, South Africa

Grignon DJ, Ro JY, Ayala AG *et al* (1992) Small cell carcinoma of the urinary bladder: a clinicopathologic analysis of 22 cases. *Cancer* **69** 527–536

Groeneveld AE, Marszalek WW and Heyns CF (1996) Bladder cancer in various population groups in the greater Durban area of KwaZulu-Natal, South Africa. *British Journal of Urology* **78** 205–208

Han R, Breitburd F, Marche PN and Orth G (1992) Linkage of regression and malignant conversion of rabbit viral papillomas to MHC class II genes. *Nature* **356** 66–68

Harnden P and Parkinson MC (1996) Transitional cell carcinoma of the bladder: diagnosis and prognosis. *Current Diagnostic Pathology* **3** 109–121

Hicks RM, James C and Webbe G (1980) Effect of *Schistosoma haematobium* and N-butyl-N-(4-hydroxybutyl)nitrosamine on the development of urothelial neoplasia in the baboon. *British Journal of Cancer* **42** 730–755

Hope-Stone HF, Oliver RTD, England HR and Blandy JP (1984) T3 bladder cancer: salvage rather than elective cystectomy after radiotherapy. *Urology* **24** 315–320

Ishak KG, Le Golvan PC and El-Sebai I (1967) Malignant bladder tumors associated with Schistosomiasis: A gross and microscopic study, In: Mostafi FK (ed). *Bilharziasis*, International Academy of Pathology Special Monograph, pp 58–83, Springer-Verlag, Berlin

Jenkins BJ, Martin JE, Baithun SI *et al* (1990) Predictions of response to radiotherapy in invasive bladder cancer. *British Journal of Urology* **65** 345–348

Kawashima M, Favre M, Obalek S, Jablonska S and Orth G (1990) Premalignant lesions and cancer of the skin in the general population: evaluation of the role of human papillomaviruses. *Journal of Investigative Dermatology* **95** 537–542

Khafagy MM, el-Bolkainy MN and Mansour MA (1972) Carcinoma of the bilharzial urinary bladder: a study of the associated mucosal lesions in 86 cases. *Cancer* **30** 150–159

Kisner CD (1973) Vesical bilharziasis, pathological changes and relationship to squamous carcinoma. *South African Journal of Surgery* **11** 79–87

Lam KY (1995) Chondroid and osseous metaplasia in carcinoma of the bladder. *Journal of Urological Pathology* **3** 255–261

Laughlin LW, Farid Z, Mansour N, Edman DC and Higashi GI (1978) Bacteriuria in urinary schistosomiasis in Egypt: a prevalence survey. *American Journal of Tropical Medical Hygiene* **27** 916–918

Makar N (1955) *Urological Aspects of Bilharziasis in Egypt*, pp 57–83, SOP Press, Cairo

Makhyoun NA, el-Kashlan KM, al-Ghorab MM and Mokhles AS (1971) Aetiological factors in bilharzial bladder cancer. *Journal of Tropical Medicine and Hygiene* **74** 73–78

Malik MO, Veress B, Daoud EH and El-Hassan AM (1975) Pattern of bladder cancer in the Sudan and its relation to schistosomiasis: a study of 255 vesical carcinomas. *Journal of Tropical Medical Hygiene* **78** 219–223

Mao EJ, Schwartz SM, Daling JR *et al* (1996) Human papilloma viruses and p53 mutations in normal pre-malignant and malignant oral epithelia. *International Journal of Cancer* **69** 152–158

Martin JE, Jenkins BJ, Zuk RJ, Blandy JP and Baithun SI (1989) Clinical importance of squamous metaplasia in invasive transitional cell carcinoma of the bladder. *Journal of Clinical Pathology* **42** 250–253

Mirvish SS (1995) Role of N-nitroso compounds (NOC) and N-nitrosation in etiology of gastric, esophageal, nasopharyngeal and bladder cancer and contribution to cancer of known exposures to NOC. *Cancer Letters* **93** 17–48

Mullokandov MR, Kholodilov NG, Atkin NB *et al* (1996) Genomic alterations in cervical carcinoma: losses of chromosome heterozygosity and human papilloma virus tumour status. *Cancer Research* **56** 197–205

Prates MD and Gillman J (1959) Carcinoma of the urinary bladder in the Portuguese East African with special reference to bilharzial cystitis and preneoplastic reactions. *South African Journal of Medical Science* **24** 13–40

Sarkis AS, Bajorin DF, Reuter VE *et al* (1995) Prognostic value of p53 nuclear overexpression in patients with invasive bladder cancer treated with neoadjuvant M-Vac. *Journal of Clinical Oncology* **13** 1384–1390

Shindoh M, Chiba I, Yasuda M *et al* (1995) Detection of human papillomavirus DNA sequence in oral squamous cell carcinomas and their relation to p53 and proliferating cell nuclear antigen expression. *Cancer* **76** 1513–1521

Snijders PJ, Scholes AG, Hart CA *et al* (1996) Prevalence of mucosotropic human papillomaviruses in squamous cell carcinoma of the head and neck. *International Journal of Cancer* **66** 464–469

Starklint H, Kjaergaard J and Jensen NK (1976) Types of metaplasia in forty urothelial bladder carcinomas: a systematic histological investigation. *Acta Pathologica Microbiologica Scandanavica* **84** 137–142

Talib H (1970) The problem of carcinoma of bilharzial bladder in Iraq. *British Journal of Urology* **42** 571–579

Vizcaino AP, Parkin DM, Boffetta P and Skinner ME (1994) Bladder cancer: epidemiology and risk factors in Bulawayo, Zimbabwe. *Cancer Causes and Control* **5** 517–522

Young RH (1996) Pathology of bladder cancer, In: Vogelzang N, Scardino P, Shipley W and Coffey D (eds). *Comprehensive Textbook of Genitourinary Oncology*, pp 326–337, Williams & Wilkins, Baltimore, Maryland

Yousem SA, Ohori NP and Sonmez-Alpan E (1992) Occurrence of human papillomavirus DNA in primary lung neoplasms. *Cancer* **69** 693–697

The authors are responsible for the accuracy of the references.

Malignancy Associated Papillomaviruses and Morphology of Human Bladder Cancer

R T D OLIVER[1] • J BREUER[2] • A M E NOURI[1] • S CAMPO[3]

[1]*Department of Oncology, St Bartholomew's Hospital, London EC1A 7BE;* [2]*Department of Virology, The Royal London Hospital, London E1 2BB;*[3]*Beatson Institute for Cancer Research, Bearsden, Glasgow G61 1BD*

Introduction
Phylogeny and taxonomy of papillomavirus
Molecular mechanisms identified from study of cancer associated papillomaviruses
Human tumours associated with HPV infection
Bovine model of papillomavirus induced cancer
HPV and bladder cancer
Potential of vaccination in papillomavirus associated cancers
Summary

INTRODUCTION

Papillomaviruses are associated with papillary tumours in many different animal species (Campo, 1997). That external factors, both genetic and environmental, can convert a benign papillomavirus induced tumour to a malignant lethal cancer is well established. The first evidence of this came from the very early studies of Shope in rabbit papillomavirus induced tumours when he showed that a benign papillary tumour virus isolated from wild rabbits could be made to produce a malignant tumour, either by painting the benign tumour with benzopyrene (Rous and Kidd, 1936) or by inoculating the virus into genetically susceptible domestic rabbits (Rous and Beard, 1935). However, the need for external co-factors is also demonstrated in those human papillomaviruses (HPV) most clearly associated with malignancy in tumours. Although HPV 16 and 18 are well established as co-factors in carcinoma of the cervix, smoking is a major co-factor in progression from premalignant to malignant disease (Daling *et al*, 1996), as is HLA phenotype (Odunsi *et al*, 1996; Davies and Stauss, 1997). The need for co-factors other than papillomavirus is also apparent in the HPV 5/8 associated squamous carcinomas occurring in patients with epidermodysplasia verruciformis. This is a rare inherited skin disorder occurring in patients with a genetic predisposition to HPV infection (Majewski and Jablonska, 1995). However, even in these patients squamous carcinomas occur only in sun exposed areas, suggesting that ultraviolet light is a critical co-factor.

Cancer Surveys Volume 31: *Bladder Cancer*
© 1998 Imperial Cancer Research Fund. 0-87969-529-3/98. $5.00 + .00

Although genetic damaging events in HPV infected cells are the best established co-factors for augmenting the transforming power of papillomaviruses, the other factor of considerable importance is immunosuppression. In addition to its DNA damaging effect, a less well recognized concomitant effect of ultra-violet light exposure is via damage to dendritic cells, which prevents antigen presentation to lymphocytes (Azizi *et al*, 1987). However, the clearest demonstration of interaction between HPV and immunosuppression in man relates to skin tumours arising in renal transplant patients on immunosuppressive drugs, of whom 65–80% were HPV positive, whereas fewer than one third of spontaneously arising tumours had detectable virus (Shamanin *et al*, 1996). Additional support for the importance of immunosuppression comes from studying ingestion of bracken as an immunosuppressive co-factor in the development of bovine papillomavirus (BPV) tumours (Jarrett *et al*, 1978), which can be rejected by use of viral protein (Campo *et al*, 1993). The report of a solitary complete remission of cervical cancer in a series of 6 patients receiving HPV 16 related E6/E7 protein vaccination provides an encouraging, albeit anecdotal, indication of the potential of this approach in human tumours (Borysiewicz *et al*, 1996).

A substantial proportion of bladder cancers have a papillary morphology (Pugh, 1973). Furthermore, there is more than one morphological variant subtype of precursor lesion (Fig. 1), suggesting that more than one papillomavirus subtype is involved. Although a few studies have looked for an association between HPV infection and bladder cancer development, the wide range of frequency, from 0 to 81% (Anwar *et al*, 1992; Wiener *et al*, 1992; Agliano *et al*, 1994; Sano *et al*, 1995), has led most authors to conclude that HPVs are not consistent co-factors in bladder cancer, or that when detected they are just passenger viruses. However, it took nearly 10 years from the first evidence that HPV might be a factor in cervical cancer until the general acceptance that HPV 16

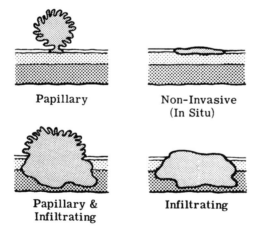

Fig. 1. Morphological classification of superficial bladder cancer (Pugh, 1973; reproduced with permission from John Wiley and Sons, Inc)

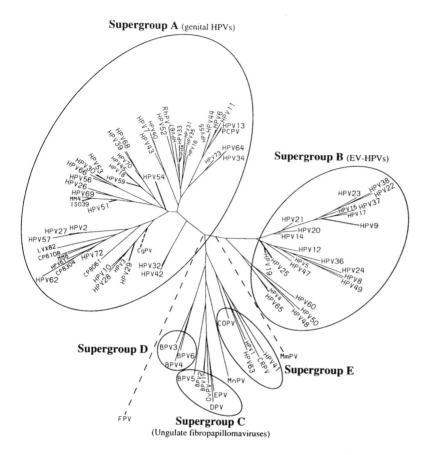

Fig. 2. A phylogenetic tree of 92 PV types based on a maximum likelihood evaluation of the 291 bp L1 segment (modified from Chan *et al*, 1995)

and 18 are major factors in that disease (zur Hausen, 1994). Furthermore, the fact that modern polymerase chain reaction (PCR) technology has identified at least 95 subtypes of HPV (Chan *et al*, 1995) means that one cannot rule out the involvement of one of the less easily identifiable viruses, as has been accepted after careful epidemiological study in skin cancers arising in immunosuppressed transplant patients (Proby *et al*, 1996). These observations and the increasing recognition of the potential for treating HPV related disease with vaccination have provided the justification for this chapter, which aims first to review in depth the mechanisms by which papillomavirus causes malignancy in bovine and human cancers, and then to examine how far the limited work on these viruses in bladder cancer supports the hypothesis that they may be more important co-factors than previously appreciated. The chapter ends by considering how the lessons from use of tumour cell vaccines in cattle could be applied to the treatment of human disease.

PHYLOGENY AND TAXONOMY OF PAPILLOMAVIRUSES

Although serology and Southern blot DNA typing have been used to identify subgroups of papillomavirus, it was the advent of PCR that led to the explosion in our knowledge of papillomavirus subtypes. Initially, when some authors reported 80% positivity in such assays on normal cervical scrapes (Young *et al*, 1989), there was a degree of scepticism as to whether false positivity might discredit use of these tests. However, with greater attention to technique, reproducible results are leading to an increasingly complex phylogenetic classification of these viruses (Chan *et al*, 1995).

The genome structure of papillomaviruses is divided into three principal regions: a long control region (LCR) and regions containing "early" (E proteins) and "late" (L proteins) genes. Papillomaviruses are classified using consensus PCR of the conserved areas of the open reading frame (ORF) of the L1 protein. The definition of a new HPV type is one that shares less than 75% homology in *L1* DNA sequences; a related HPV subtype is defined as one that shares at least 75% though less than 90% homology in *L1* DNA sequences. Chan *et al* (1995) reviewed genomic sequences of 95 papillomavirus types based on a 291 base pair segment of the *L1* gene and concluded that there were five phylogenetically distinct subgroups (Fig. 2). Two (types A and B) predominated in humans, the genital/mucocutaneous group mainly associated with anogenital and oral cancer and the epidermodysplasia verruciformis group involved in skin pathology. The subtypes produce a variety of different tumours, ranging from the benign verruca picked up by most children after their first visit to public swimming pools to malignant squamous carcinomas of the skin. They are particularly prevalent in tumours arising in organ transplant recipients on long term immunosuppression. The third and fourth subtypes (types C and D) were found in cattle, and the fifth (E) consisted of a mixture of human as well as canine and rabbit subtypes.

MOLECULAR MECHANISMS IDENTIFIED FROM STUDY OF CANCER ASSOCIATED PAPILLOMAVIRUSES

The life cycle of papillomaviruses (for review see Campo, 1997) is tightly coupled to epithelial cell maturation and differentiation: the virus infects the basal keratinocytes, expresses some of its genes in the basal and suprabasal layers, replicates its genome in the differentiating spinous and granular layers and expresses its structural genes and packages its DNA in the squamous layers. New infectious virus is finally released with the desquamation of the keratinized squames (Fig. 3). Occasionally, benign warts may persist and progress to squamous carcinoma. However, neoplastic progression is a dead end process for the virus, because the transformed cell loses the ability to permit virus maturation and can even lose the papillomavirus DNA altogether in a form of "hit and run" transformation process (Campo *et al*, 1985), something which can also be

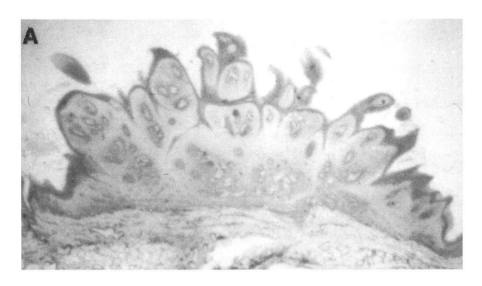

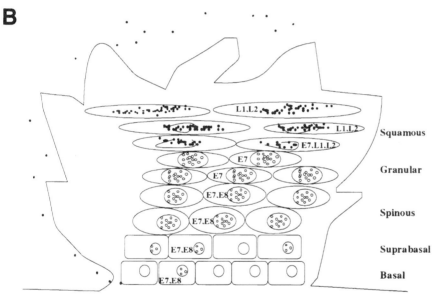

Fig. 3. (A) Section of a typical oesophageal papilloma (haematoxylin and eosin x 10). (B) Schematic representation of a papilloma and of the life cycle of papillomavirus. Viral DNA is represented by small open circles and virions by small filled circles. The localization of the BPV 4 proteins E7, E8, L1 and L2 is indicated. (For reference see Campo, in press)

demonstrated in experimental tumour induction studies using chemical immunosuppressive drugs and viral inoculation. However, more usually the DNA is either incorporated into the cellular DNA or maintained as an extra-chromosomal element (which replicates in synchrony with the cell cycle) but never leads to productive virus, which explains why fully formed virus is never detected in associated tumours.

Although this cell cycle has been worked out in detail for one of the less malignant papillomaviruses, it is reasonable to assume that most viruses behave in a similar way unless the circumstances permit actual cell transformation. This is facilitated either by sufficient immunosuppression to enable continued proliferation, a host genetic environment of low immune response or high susceptibility to the cell cycle influencing effects of the papillomavirus proteins, or by mutational damage from environmental carcinogens. Any of these processes, by facilitating the critical steps of early transformation, ultimately facilitates malignant progression, because of the continuous proliferation facilitated by the early changes.

Although papillomaviruses in general are not highly transforming when cultured in vitro some, particularly the high risk mucosal types associated with cervical cancer, are more active in these assays than the others (Vousden, 1994). Although many of the genes within the papillomavirus genome have a part in facilitating host cell proliferation, two seem to play a particularly important role, particularly in the high risk mucosal subgroup, type A (Fig. 2), of which HPV 16 and 18 are the prototypes. The two critical proteins are E6 and E7. E6, as well as activating telomerase to block the normal clock of cell ageing and promote cell immortalization, also causes a direct inhibition of the activity of TP53. This protein, when normally functional, has a critical role in initiating apoptosis of any cell with a mutation that cannot be repaired by DNA enzymes (Lane, 1992). The importance of this particular protein in the transforming activity of HPV 16/18 in cervical cancer is emphasized by the observation that the minority of cervical cancers that are HPV negative have a very high prevalence of *TP53* mutations, whereas those that are virus positive very rarely have such defects (Fujita *et al*, 1992; Busby-Earle *et al*, 1994). HPV 16/18 E7 has an equally important effect in that it blocks another tumour suppressor protein RB (the retinoblastoma susceptibility gene product). Although these molecular pathways are well demonstrated for HP16/18, such mechanisms are thought to be less active in the supergroup B (epidermodysplasia verruciformis) viruses. These viruses have developed other transforming mechanisms, such as that associated with E2. BPV subtypes, particularly supergroup D, do not have an *E6* gene, and a co-operation between *E7* and *E8* is thought to be the critical event in transformation.

One other molecular mechanism involved in malignant transformation by papillomaviruses has been identified in both HPV 16 and bovine papillomavirus infected cells. This is that the viral protein E5, or its homologue E8, as well as facilitating anchorage independent growth and causing disruption of gap junction intercellular communications (Faccini *et al*, 1996), can also upregulate epithelial growth factor receptor (EGFR) by blocking its breakdown and increasing its recycling from endosomal compartments (Straight *et al*, 1995). As upregulated EGFR is a common risk factor for increased malignancy in many adult solid cancers (Nouri *et al*, 1995), particularly bladder, head and neck and cervical cancer, this observation provides another reason to justify study of papillomaviruses in bladder cancer.

One aspect of HPV induced cervical cancer that has not been extensively investigated is the degree of chromosomal alterations that are induced in association with clonal progression to invasion and metastasis, as has been done so extensively in colon cancer (Vogelstein *et al*, 1989) and bladder cancer (Dalbagni *et al*, 1993). In experimental bovine papillomavirus induced upper alimentary cancer, there have been interesting studies of the interaction between BPV 4 and the flavonoid quercetin, which is one of the principal mutagenic substances that can be isolated from bracken. Cairney and Campo (1995) have demonstrated that in quercetin treated BPV infected cells *E7* is the only BPV 4 oncogene required for full transformation, because the chemical substitutes for *E8* in conferring anchorage independence—for *E6* in inducing immortalization and for mutant TP53 in inducing tumorigenesis. Despite this, quercetin treated fully transformed tumour cells seldom have *TP53* mutations. One possible explanation is that quercetin upregulates the transcription activity of the BPV 4 LCR through a cis activating element. Given the importance of transcriptional thresholds in cell transformation, this is thought to be a mechanism by which quercetin enhances malignant progression of BPV infected cells (Campo, 1997).

HUMAN TUMOURS ASSOCIATED WITH HPV INFECTION

Although cervix (zur Hausen, 1994) and non-melanoma skin cancers (Proby *et al*, 1996) have been the human tumours most clearly associated with a specific human papillomavirus infection, carcinoma of the anus (zur Hausen, 1991) and penis (Daling *et al*, 1994) are also clearly associated. Surprisingly given its squamous morphology, relatively little work has been done on the role of papillomavirus in oral squamous cancers (Yeudall and Campo, 1991; Shindoh *et al*, 1995).

Providing important evidence of the role of immune surveillance in prevention of papillomavirus tumours is the extremely high incidence of cervix (Maiman *et al*, 1997) and anal carcinoma (Schulz *et al*, 1996) in HIV infected individuals. The association of HIV infection with treatment resistant premalignant cervical cancer is so strong that it has been incorporated as one of the diagnostic features of an AIDS defining illness, which contrasts with the rarity with which male homosexuals mention the risk of anal carcinoma after HIV infection. Surprisingly, there is as yet no increase in the incidence of penile cancer in HIV infected individuals, possibly because in the west it is a disease of the elderly. In addition, as circumcision is so widely practised in the USA, hygiene probably prevents this becoming a problem. More interesting statistics may emerge from the areas of central Africa and Brazil where circumcision is not routine and the incidence of cancer of the penis is among the highest in the world in non-immunosuppressed men. Although there are no detailed statistics available as yet to answer this question, anecdotal experience (R.T.D.O.) of an HIV positive patient in Kenya who went through puberty at age 11 and died from fulminating carcinoma of the penis at age 16 suggests that there could be some justification for trying to find out the global statistics on this disease.

The first suggestion of an association between HPV and carcinoma of the cervix came from zur Hausen (Lopez-Beltran *et al*, 1996) after it was reported that condyloma acuminata was associated with a "benign" papillomavirus. Over a period of 10 years the medical profession remained very sceptical that HPV was anything more than an innocent passenger virus. However, as discussed in the previous section, with the uncovering of the complex genetic mechanisms involving *E6/E7* that are involved in transformation, taken with the epidemiological evidence (Tables 1 and 2) it can now be little disputed that HPV infection is a major but by no means an absolute determinant of the disease, given the 10% HPV negative tumours and 30% incidence of positivity in young healthy men.

That smoking is a critical co-factor with HPV in cervical cancer is clearly established (Daling *et al*, 1996), although the observation that the husband's smoking habit is also a factor (Table 3) (Zunzunegui *et al*, 1986) again raises the question of how much the immunosuppressive effect of semen or continued intercourse with the man who was the source of HPV infection contributes. With evidence that use of barrier contraception for 6 months is associated with 100% incidence of spontaneous regression of cervical intraepithelial neoplasia III (Richardson and Lyon, 1981), there is increasing interest in the earlier studies on the immunosuppressive effect of semen (Read *et al*, 1978). These authors showed considerable variation in the suppressive effect of semen within the male population but did not attempt to correlate the degree of immunosuppression with extent of smoking. Evidence that immunosuppression is one side effect of heavy smoking that could increase the persistence of HPV in men who smoke and could explain the association by a mechanism other than its mutagenic effect comes from a small study in women with cervical cancer which showed that smokers with cervical cancer had a lower CD4/CD8 ratio than non-smokers (Kesic *et al*, 1993). Additional understanding about how the disease develops comes from the studies of HLA antigen frequency (Table 4). To date 10 of 12 studies have shown an association with class II HLA DQB1°03. This observation is thought to be mediated via altered T lymphocyte response to HPV antigens and emphasizes the importance of host genetics in expression of the malignant effect of HPV in the causation of cervical cancer (Davies and Stauss, 1997; Odunsi *et al*, 1996).

As far as skin cancer is concerned, there is little debate that epidermodysplasia verruciformis is associated principally with HPV 5 and HPV 8 in more than 90% of individuals with the disease (Majewski and Jablonska, 1995) and that the strength of the association equals or exceeds that seen between HPV 16 and 18 and cervical cancer. Epidermodysplasia verruciformis is an inherited

TABLE 1. HPV in normal and malignant cervical scraps[a]

	No tested	Proportion HPV
"Normals" <35 y old	3048	17%
"Normals" ≥35 y old	3172	5.3%
Cervical cancer	557	93%

[a]Modified from Brule *et al* (1993)

TABLE 2. HPV subtypes in cervical cancer[a]

	No tested	Total positive	HPV 16	HPV 18	Other types	Unclassified
USA	29	100%	76%	17%	7%	nil
USA	153	89%	47%	24%	10%	5.2%
Netherlands	120	100%	73%	8%	2.5%	5.8%
France	106	84%	55%	12%	6.6%	10%
East Africa	53	89%	38%	32%	5.7%	13.2%
India	96	98%	64%	3.1%	1%	30%

[a]Modified from Brule *et al* (1993)

TABLE 3. Risk factors for cervical cancer in married hispanic women[a]

Risk factor	Odds ratio	p value
Husband had >20 partners	5.3	<0.01
Husband current or past smoker	3.3	<0.07
Wife's number of sexual partners	1.0	0.90
Wife's age at 1st intercourse	2.0	<0.03

[a]Modified from Zunzunegui *et al* (1986)

condition that presents with multiple warts on various body sites with average onset of warts at age 6, although skin cancers do not develop for an average of 24.5 years. Since they occur almost exclusively in sun exposed skin, it is clear that this disease shows the typical behaviour of an HPV related cancer, that is depending on interacting co-factors, in this case mutagenesis and immunosuppression from ultraviolet light before the life threatening phenotype is expressed. The occurrence of an increased frequency of epidermodysplasia verruciformis related HPV subtypes in non-melanoma skin cancers developing after transplant demonstrates this same interdependence of co-factors. These skin cancers occur in up to 44% of organ transplant recipients, taking 10–25 years after transplant to develop (Table 5).

Despite this plethora of HPV types detected in epidermodysplasia verruciformis patients and in tumours arising in immunosuppressed individuals, most

TABLE 4. HLV class II antigen studies in cervix cancer[a]

Wank and Thomssen (1991)	DQ3
Wank *et al* (1992)	$DQB_1°0303$
Wank *et al* (1993)	$DQB_1°0303$
Gregoire *et al* (1993)	$DQB_1°0303$
	$DQB_1°0604$
Nawa *et al* (1995)	$DQB_1°0301$
	$DQB_1°0303$
Helland *et al* (1994)	$DQB_1°03$
Saste-Garau *et al* (1996)	$DQB_1°03$
Vandenvelde *et al* (1993)	(+DQB°03 in CIN)
Glew *et al* (1993)	—
Duggan-Keen *et al* (1996)	—
Apple *et al* (1995)	(+DQB°03 in CIN)
Odunsi *et al* (1995, 1996)	($DQB_1°03$ C+DQB°03 in CIN)

[a]For reference, see Davies and Stauss (1997)

studies in spontaneously arising skin cancers show a very low incidence (Table 5). Two exceptions to this are those rare tumours arising adjacent to the finger nails and on the palms or soles (periungual and palmoplantar squamous cell carcinoma and Bowen's disease), where the frequency of HPV 16 has been in excess of 60%. The finding that some of these cases had HPV 16 infection of skin and cervix suggests that genital transmission via the fingers might be a factor (Proby *et al*, 1996).

The overall low HPV positivity in the common spontaneously occurring squamous skin carcinoma raises the question as to how far Campo's observation of "hit and run," with virus initiating the benign phase of tumour growth but with no virus sequences persisting after malignant transformation, is a factor (Campo *et al*, 1985). That this may not be the total explanation comes from the report

TABLE 5. HPV DNA in cutaneous squamous cell carcinoma[a]

No of studies	No of cases	Total proportion HPV positive	Proportion specific HPV[b]	Range
3+	242	0.8%	0.4%	0–5%
3+	65	25%	12%	18–33%
6+	188	69%	36%	60–81%
Total IS tumours[c]	495	30%	16%	
Control tissues[c]	56	18%	7%	0–32%
SCC[d]	76	3%	3%	—
BCC[d]	53	2%	2%	—
SCC/BCC[e]	40	35%	ND	—

[a]Modified from Proby *et al* (1996)
[b]Common cutaneous, common mucosal or HPV 5/8
[c]Immunosuppressed transplant recipient tumours or control tissues
[d]Spontanenous tumours (Kawashima *et al*, 1990)
[e]Spontaneous tumours (Shamanin *et al*, 1996)

that when less stringent levels of PCR homology are screened by using "degenerate" PCR detection methods, HPV DNA can be identified in 35% of spontaneous skin cancers, suggesting that rarer or as yet undefined HPV may be involved (Shamanin *et al*, 1996).

BOVINE MODEL OF PAPILLOMAVIRUS INDUCED CANCER

Bovine papillomaviruses fall into two groups, supergroups C and D in Fig. 2. The BPV members of the first supergroup are known as fibropapillomaviruses (BPV 1, 2 and 5), because they initially transform the subepithelial fibroblasts before going on to cause epithelial plexiform acanthosis and then papillomatosis (Jarrett, 1985), whereas the viruses of the second supergroup, the epitheliotrophic papillomaviruses (BPV 3, 4 and 6), cause epithelial papillomas (Jarrett *et al*, 1984). BPV 1 causes teat frond and penile fibropapillomas, whereas BPV 2 is the agent of common cutaneous warts but is also associated with both naturally occurring and experimental bladder cancer. BPV 5 causes rice grain fibropapillomas of the udder. BPV 3 is associated with cutaneous lesions, whereas BPV 4 is the principal agent associated with upper alimentary tumours, including oral cancers, and shows considerable target specificity when inoculated in experimental studies, causing tumours only when in alimentary canal epithelium but not in skin (Jarrett *et al*, 1984). BPV 6 has been primarily associated with teat papillomas (Jarrett *et al*, 1984).

In healthy cattle the papillomas at all these sites normally regress totally. However, in regions where there is a high level of bracken fern (*Pteridium aquilinum*), which contains both carcinogens (Evans *et al*, 1984) and immunosuppressants (Evans *et al*, 1982), there is persistent papillomatosis, and a higher proportion of papillomas progress to cancer (Plowright *et al*, 1971; Jarrett *et al*, 1978; Jackson *et al*, 1993).

Bracken fed cattle become chronically immunosuppressed and develop bladder tumours (which manifest by causing haematuria) and alimentary canal cancers (which manifest by causing vomiting) (Plowright *et al*, 1971; Jarrett *et al*, 1978). The findings in one study that bracken exposed animals had a high incidence of chromosomal abnormalities in their lymphocytes (Moura *et al*, 1988) demonstrate that there may be additional factors to immunosuppression involved. The association of BPV and cancer has been confirmed by induction of the same diseases in cattle inoculated experimentally with BPV and fed bracken (Campo *et al*, 1992, 1994b).

Bracken feeding causes two marked haematological effects. Acute high dose causes a fall in polymorphs and death from septicaemia, whereas lower doses fed chronically cause lymphopenia, which is very slow to recover after bracken withdrawal. In an attempt to distinguish between the immunosuppressive and mutagenic properties of bracken, a study was done on animals treated with azathioprine, a drug normally used in suppressing immune response of transplant recipients. Even without experimental inoculation of BPV, bladder tumours developed in the immunosuppressed animals (Campo *et al*, 1992). The transitional cell tumours that developed were indistinguishable from the naturally occurring ones, although in addition some animals developed haemangioendotheliomas of the adjacent capillaries, on their own or in association with transitional cell cancer. Although morphologically the experimental tumours were little different from the normal counterparts, they showed less evidence of malignant transformation into invasive and metastatic disease. Despite this, 69% of the tumours were BPV 2 positive, compared with 46% of the spontaneous tumours. Although this suggests that immunosuppression may be sufficient on its own to activate latent papillomaviruses, it must be remembered that azathioprine itself is mutagenic, and so for definitive proof it would be necessary to extend these studies to animals treated with anti-lymphocyte globulin and/or cyclosporin A.

One unexpected finding from these experiments was that immunosuppression on its own was capable of uncovering latent infection of both BPV 2 in the bladder and also BPV 1 or BPV 2 in skin warts. In immunocompetent calves skin warts seemed to occur only at sites of skin damage (Campo *et al*, 1994a), supporting views published from other papillomavirus studies (Siegsmund *et al*, 1991) that trauma or chronic mechanical irritation is a way of activating latent papillomavirus. As well as providing a caution to urologists using extensive diathermy in the treatment of their patients, this mechanism could also be extended to explain the high incidence of HPV associated anal carcinoma in male homosexuals who participate in anal intercourse, which is often associated with bleeding.

One other aspect of considerable practical importance from the point of view of studying HPV in bladder cancer is that BPV DNA can be detected in the peripheral blood lymphocytes of animals with BPV associated bladder tumours (Campo *et al*, 1994a). Reports that lymphocytes from HPV infected cervical cancer patients are also positive for HPV DNA (Kedzia *et al*, 1992) would also support this view.

HPV AND BLADDER CANCER

As mentioned in the introduction, evidence for involvement of HPV in bladder cancer is far from certain. Table 6 summarizes 15 literature reports of 719 tumours that have been typed, with 19% positive overall, ranging from 0 to 81%. Because the two largest series have been either totally negative or of a very low frequency, and the most recent positive study showed equal frequency in normal and malignant tissue (Table 7), the general consensus is that the common HPVs are not as actively involved as in cervical cancer and are being picked up as contaminants because these tissues are the "normal" reservoir for such viruses. However, as this observation means that HPVs may be present for the whole life cycle of bladder tumours, there remains the possibility that the concept of "hit and run" (Campo *et al*, 1985) may be tenable, as has been shown

TABLE 6. Overview of HPVB studies in human bladder cancer

No of studies	No of cases tested	% Positive	Range
5[a]	248	0	
3[b]	142	6%	(2–9%)
3[c]	119	17%	(16–20%)
4[d]	204	53%	(29–81%)
Total	713	19	(0–81%)

[a]Ostrow et al, 1987; Knowles, 1992; Saltzstein et al, 1993; Sinclair et al, 1993; Sano et al, 1995
[b]Bryant et al, 1991; Kerley et al, 1991; Lopez-Beltran et al, 1996
[c]Chetsanga et al, 1992; Shibutani et al, 1992; Ludwig et al, 1996
[d]Anwar et al, 1992; Rotola et al, 1992; Furihata et al, 1993; Agliano et al, 1994

in the bovine model. The striking difference in frequency of HPV in spontaneous and immunosuppressed skin cancers (Table 5) would support the view that the "hit and run" hypothesis may be a mechanism whereby HPVs cause cancer in men and might be involved in bladder cancer. Screening tumours by E6, E7 and LCR sequences could provide evidence to support this view. A final alternative is that there are other papillomavirus subtypes that are specific for bladder cancer but have not yet been tested.

Our own interest in HPV in bladder cancer began when we observed a young woman kidney transplant recipient who had married an older man after being on immunosuppression for 6 months and who developed florid vulval warts and haematuria. Cystoscopy revealed tumours in the urethra and bladder that had the typical macroscopic morphology of conventional transitional cell tumours. Histology revealed transitional cell with squamous metaplasia, and typing the tumour for HPV revealed HPV11 (Rovere *et al*, 1988). The disease, having recurred after transurethreal resection, cleared after 12 months' treatment with interferon and has remained clear for more than 10 years. A second case

TABLE 7. HPV in normal control v bladder cancer tissues

Reference	Normal control tissues	Bladder cancer tissues
Anwar et al (1992)	33% (n=21)	81% (n=48)
Rotola et al (1992)	88% (n=8)	77% (n=26)
Agliano et al (1994)	0% (n=10)	50% (n=46)
Ludwig et al (1996)	19% (n=23)	19% (n=23)
Total	29% (n=62)	60% (n=143)

occurred in an unmarried patient not on immunosuppressive drugs but with cutaneous type papillary tumours on the vulva, urethra and in the bladder. However, no tissue was available for viral studies. Also, a small study of women with recurrent urethral syndrome who had positive biopsies for HPV in the urethra (Philp T, personal communication) provided reasonable evidence that papillomavirus, like bacteria such as *Escherichia coli*, can progress from the vulva to the bladder via the urethra, at least in the female. With reports of condyloma acuminata being demonstrated in the bladder and one case in which progression from benign condyloma to malignant cancer was documented (Wilson *et al*, 1990), it seemed reasonable to conclude that proof of principle had been established.

Although screening bladder cancers for HPV has been predominantly negative to date, the results are little different from the frequency reported in spontaneous skin cancer using similar assays (Table 5). Given this observation, screening needs to be extended to other HPV types and, as was done with skin cancers, should include screening with "degenerate" primers to attempt to detect cross reactivity with related viruses. In an initial screen using L1 ORF primers, GP5/6 and MYO9/11, we had conflicting results in that neither gave any reaction with a mixed group of 14 bladder and prostate cancers or 9 bladder cell lines at the standard temperature of 55°C, but all of the samples reacted and gave a 450bp band suggesting HPV infection at 40°C with MY09/11 but not with GP5/6. As this band was also developed, without sequencing, by other human cells but not a baboon tissue control, without doing sequencing it is unclear how specific this reaction was for an oncogenic virus (Sinclair *et al*, 1993).

Currently we are attempting to take this research further using an additional group of "degenerative" primers, including markers for all of the supergroups identified in Fig. 2.

POTENTIAL OF VACCINATION IN PAPILLOMAVIRUS ASSOCIATED CANCERS

The single "anecdotal" report of complete regression of established recurrence from cervical cancer following vaccination with recombinant E6 and E7 protein from HPV 16 in a series of 6 patients treated as part of a phase I study (Borysiewicz *et al*, 1996) raises a question as to whether there may be potential for use of HPV vaccines as therapy in patients with measurable disease, rather than focusing totally on adjuvant studies. This is despite perceived wisdom from studies in experimental animals that cancer vaccines are better explored in minimal residual disease. Personal involvement (R.T.D.O.) in an adjuvant vaccine programme for leukaemia using allogeneic tumour cells that took 8 years to prove the principle wrong (Powles *et al*, 1977)—one reason for the failure possibly having been that the tumour rejection antigen was self MHC restricted (Lee and Oliver, 1978; Oliver and Lee, 1979)—indicates that a measurable disease model has considerable advantage in terms of speed of progress. As it has been known that regressor versus progressor phenotype in animal models of papillomavirus induced tumour is influenced by immune status, it might be preferable for HPV vaccine studies to be focused on patients with measurable disease in order to get the dose and scheduling correct before rushing to do adjuvant trials.

Support for the view that more work is justified in the setting of measurable disease comes from study of papillomavirus vaccination in cattle. Long before purified BPV proteins or even pure viral preparations were available, vets learned that it was possible to induce tumour rejection using crude suspensions of tumour cells (Hoffmann *et al*, 1981). Given the success of the marker tumour studies in patients with superficial bladder cancer using BCG (Lamm, 1995), whole tumour extract studies could be justified in bladder cancer today even without identifying a specific HPV involvement. It is possible that using a virus of low pathogenicity, such as Newcastle disease virus, to produce a viral oncolysate, as was first used by Lindenmann (Lindenmann and Klein, 1967) in animals, might make such an approach in patients with measurable superficial disease extremely interesting and might even be tried in patients with metastases.

For the future, however, it will be important to focus on the attempts to do studies using purified proteins or whole virus. In the cattle model whole viruses have been shown to work successfully (Campo and Jarrett, 1994), with long lasting resistance being immunologically specific in that rechallenge with another type invariably produced a new infection. More recent studies have focused on subunit vaccines based on the structural proteins BPV 2 L1 and L2 as well as BPV 4 L2 and E7. Protection was demonstrated using L1 and L2, more significantly with L2. The E7 vaccine was less active even when measured in assays of early regression of established warts. Vaccination protection has also been shown using L2 in rabbits. In cattle the N-terminus of L2 is sufficient for full protection and there is some evidence of homology between the immunodominant epitope of bovine L2 and that of several genital HPVs (Kawashima *et al*, 1990; Brule *et al*, 1993; Campo and Jarrett, 1994; Chandrachud *et al*, 1995; Kirnbauer *et al*, 1996; Campo, 1997).

SUMMARY

Animal studies in rabbit and cattle have clearly demonstrated the contribution of host genetics, chemical carcinogens and immunosuppression to the conversion of papillomavirus induced benign regressing warts into malignant cancers. More significant is the role of vaccination both with whole tumour cell suspensions with whole virus and viral proteins, particularly L2 molecules, in causing progressing warts to regress. Early results in small scale studies of HPV16 E6/E7 vaccine in patients with cervical cancer have provided evidence that tumour regression can be induced in human papillomavirus induced tumours.

These observations provided added impetus for more research to firm up the increasing, but still principally anecdotal, evidence that papillomaviruses may be involved in the pathogenesis of bladder cancer. Studies of carcinomas arising in cattle after BBV 4 infection show absence of fully infectious virus in the majority of tumours, though the tumours have persistent *E7*, *E8* and LCR sequences. As this is all that is required for transformation, it may require in vitro molecular studies in human bladder cancer screening for such elements before final proof of involvement is confirmed. However, even before this is achieved, given the success in animal models of whole tumour cell vaccines, serious thought should be given to how to develop protocols for study of crude tumour cell vaccines in vivo. Such studies would need in vitro assays to seek evidence for specific antitumour immunity, focusing on studies of tumour infiltrating lymphocytes and their T cell receptor polymorphisms.

References

Agliano AM, Gradilone A, Gazzaniga P *et al* (1994) High frequency of human papillomavirus detection in urinary bladder cancer. *Urologia Internationalis* **53** 125–129

Anwar K, Naiki H, Nakakuki K and Inuzuka M (1992) High frequency of human papillomavirus infection in carcinoma of the urinary bladder. *Cancer* **70** 1967–1973

Azizi E, Bucana C, Goldberg L and Kripke L (1987) Perturbation of epidermal Langerhans cells in basal cell carcinomas. *American Journal of Dermatology* **9** 6465–6473

Borysiewicz L, Fiander A, Nimako M *et al* (1996) A recombinant vaccinia virus encoding human papillomavirus type-16 and type-18, E6 and E7 proteins as immunotherapy for cervical cancer. *Lancet* **347** 1523–1527

Brule AVD, Snijders P, Meijer C and Walboomers J (1993) PCR-based detection of genital HPV genotypes: an update and future perspectives. *Papillomavirus Reports* **4** 95–99

Bryant P, Davies P and Wilson D (1991) Detection of human papillomavirus DNA in cancer of the urinary bladder by in situ hybridisation. *British Journal of Urology* **68** 49–52

Busby-Earle RM, Steel CM, Williams AR, Cohen B and Bird CC (1994) p53 mutations in cervical carcinogenesis: low frequency and lack of correlation with human papillomavirus status. *British Journal of Cancer* **69** 732–737

Cairney M and Campo M (1995) The synergism between bovine papillomavirus type 4 and quercetin is dependent on the timing of exposure. *Carcinogenesis* **16** 1997–2001

Campo MS (1997) Bovine papilloma virus and cancer. *British Veterinary Journal* **154** 175–188

Campo M and Jarrett W (1994) Vaccination against cutaneous and mucosal papillomavirus in cattle, In: Chadwick DJ and Marsh J (eds). *Vaccines Against Virally Induced Cancers* (Ciba Foundation Symposium no 187) 61–77, Wiley, Chichester

Campo MS, Moar MH, Sartirana ML, Kennedy IM and Jarrett WF (1985) The presence of bovine papillomavirus type 4 DNA is not required for the progression to, or the maintenance of, the malignant state in cancers of the alimentary canal in cattle. *EMBO Journal* **4** 1819–1825

Campo M, Jarrett W, Barron R, O'Neil B and Smith K (1992) Association of bovine papillomavirus type 2 and bracken fern with bladder cancer in cattle. *Cancer Research* **52** 6898–6904

Campo M, Grindlay G, O'Neil B *et al* (1993) Prophylactic and therapeutic vaccination against a mucosal papillomavirus. *Journal of General Virology* **74** 945–953

Campo M, Jarrett W, O'Neil B and Barron R (1994a) Latent papillomavirus infection in cattle. *Research in Veterinary Science* **56** 151–157

Campo M, O'Neil B, Barron R and Jarrett W (1994b) Experimental reproduction of the papilloma-carcinoma complex of the alimentary canal in cattle. *Carcinogenesis* **15** 1597–1601

Chan S-Y, Delius H, Halpern A and Bernard HU (1995) Analysis of genomic sequences of 95 papillomavirus types: uniting typing, phylogeny and taxonomy. *Journal of Virology* **69** 3074–3083

Chandrachud L, Grindlay G, McGarvie G *et al* (1995) Vaccination of cattle with the N-terminus of L2 is necessary and sufficient for preventing infection by bovine papillomavirus-4. *Virology* **211** 204–208

Chetsanga C, Malmstrom PU, Gyllensten U *et al* (1992) Low incidence of human papillomavirus type 16 DNA in bladder tumor detected by the polymerase chain reaction. *Cancer* **69** 1208–1211

Dalbagni G, Presti G, Reuter J, Fair W and Cordon-Cardo C (1993) Genetic alterations in bladder cancer. *Lancet* **342** 469–471

Daling J, Madeleine M, Sherman K, Beckmann A and Gregory-Hislop T (eds) (1994) *Accomplishments in Cancer Research*, pp 280–287, JP Lippincot Co, Philadelphia, Pennsylvania

Daling JR, Madeleine MM, McKnight B *et al* (1996) The relationship of human papillomavirus-related cervical tumors to cigarette smoking, oral contraceptive use, and prior herpes simplex virus type 2 infection. *Cancer Epidemiology Biomarkers and Prevention* **5** 541–548

Davies DH and Stauss H (1997) The significance of human leukocyte antigen associations with cervical cancer. *Papillomavirus Report* **8** 43–50

Evans I, Prorok J, Cole R *et al* (1984) The carcinogenic, mutagenic and teratogenic toxicity of bracken. *Proceedings of the Royal Society of Edinburgh* **81** 65–77

Evans W, Patel M and Koohy Y (1982) Acute bracken poisoning in homogastric and ruminant animals. *Proceedings of the Royal Society of Edinburgh* **81** 29–64

Faccini AM, Cairney M, Ashrafi GH *et al* (1996) The bovine papillomavirus type 4 E8 protein binds to ductin and causes loss of gap junctional intercellular communication in primary fibroblasts. *Journal of Virology* **70** 9041–9045

Fujita M, Inoue M, Tanizawa O, Iwamoto S and Enomoto T (1992) Alterations of the p53 gene in human primary cervical carcinoma with and without human papillomavirus infection. *Cancer Research* **52** 5323–5328

Furihata M, Inoue K, Ohtsuki Y *et al* (1993) High-risk human papillomavirus infections and overexpression of p53 protein as prognostic indicators in transitional cell carcinoma of the urinary bladder. *Cancer Research* **53** 4823–4827

Hoffmann D, Jennings P and Spradbrow P (1981) Immunotherapy of bovine ocular squamous cell carcinomas with phenol-saline extracts of allogeneic carcinomas. *Australian Veterinarian Journal* **57** 159–163

Jackson M, Campo M and Gaukroger J (1993) Cooperation between papillomavirus and chemical cofactors in oncogenesis. *Clinical Reviews of Oncology* **4** 277–291

Jarrett W (1985) The natural history of bovine papillomavirus infections. *Advances in Viral Oncology* **5** 83–102

Jarrett W, McNeil P, Grimshaw W, Selman I and McIntyre W (1978) High incidence area of cattle cancer with a possible interaction between an environmental carcinogen and a papilloma virus. *Nature* **274** 215–217

Jarrett W, Campo M, O'Neil B, Laird H and Coggins L (1984) A novel bovine papillomavirus (BPV6) causing true epithelial papillomas of the mammary gland skin: a member of a proposed new BPV subgroup. *Virology* **136** 255–264

Kawashima M, Favre M, Obalek S, Jablonska S and Orth G (1990) Premalignant lesions and cancer of the skin in the general population: evaluation of the role of human papillomaviruses. *Journal of Investigative Dermatology* **95** 537–542

Kedzia H, Gozdzicka-Jozefiak A, Wolna M and Tomczak E (1992) Distribution of human papillomavirus 16 in the blood of women with uterine cervix carcinoma. *European Journal of Gynaecological Oncology* **6** 522–526

Kerley SW, Persons DL and Fishback JL (1991) Human papillomavirus and carcinoma of the urinary bladder. *Modern Pathology* **4** 316–319

Kesic V, Jevremovic M, Petkovic S and Arsenovic N (1993) T4/T8 lymphocyte ratio related to smoking habits in patients with cancer of the uterine cervix. *European Journal of Cancer* **29a** **(Supplement 6)** [Abstract 713]

Kirnbauer R, Chandrachuud L, O'Neil B *et al* (1996) Virus-like particles of bovine papillomavirus type 4 in prophylactic and therapeutic immunization. *Virology* **218** 37–44

Knowles MA (1992) Human papillomavirus sequences are not detectable by Southern blotting or general primer-mediated polymerase chain reaction in transitional cell tumours of the bladder. *Urological Research* **20** 297–301

Lamm D (1995) BCG in perspective: advances in the treatment of superficial bladder cancer. *European Urology* **27** 2–8

Lane DP (1992) p53, guardian of the genome. *Nature* **358** 15–16

Lee SK and Oliver RTD (1978) Autologous leukaemia specific T-cell mediated lymphotoxicity in patients with acute myelogous leukaemia. *Journal of Experimental Medicine* **147** 912–922

Lindenmann J and Klein PA (1967) Viral oncolysis: increased immunogenicity of host cell antigen associated with influenza virus. *Journal of Experimental Medicine* **126** 93–108

Lopez-Beltran A, Escudero AL, Vicioso L, Munoz E and Carrasco JC (1996) Human papillomavirus DNA as a factor determining the survival of bladder cancer patients. *British Journal of Cancer* **73** 124–127

Ludwig M, Kochel HG, Fischer C, Ringert RH and Weidner W (1996) Human papillomavirus in tissue of bladder and bladder carcinoma specimens: a preliminary study. *European Urology* **30** 96–102

Maiman M, Fruchter R, Clark M *et al* (1997) Cervical cancer as an AIDS-defining illness. *Obstetrics and Gynecology* **89** 76–80

Majewski S and Jablonska S (1995) Epidermodysplasia verruciformis as a model of human papillomavirus-induced genetic cancer of the skin. *Archives of Dermatology* **131** 1312–1318

Moura J, Stocco-dos-Santos R, Daglki M *et al* (1988) Chromosome aberrations in cattle raised on bracken fern pasture. *Experientia* **44** 785–788

Nouri A, Hussain R and Oliver R (1995) Epidermal growth factor induced protection of tumour cell susceptibility to cytolosis. *European Journal of Cancer* **31** 963–969

Odunsi K, Terry G, Ho L *et al* (1996) Susceptibility to human papillomavirus-associated cervical intra-epithelial neoplasia is determined by specific HLA DR-DQ alleles. *International Journal of Cancer* **67** 595–602

Oliver RTD and Lee SK (eds) (1979) Self-restricted cytotoxicity against myeloid leukaemia cells, In: Riethmuller G, Wernet P and Cudkowicz G (eds). *Natural and Induced Cell-Mediated Cytotoxicity*, pp 183–189, Academic Press, New York

Ostrow RS, Manias DA, Fong WJ, Zachow KR and Faras AJ (1987) A survey of human cancers for human papillomavirus DNA by filter hybridization. *Cancer* **59** 429–434

Plowright W, Linsell C and Peers F (1971) A focus of rumenal cancer in Kenyan cattle. *British Journal of Cancer* **25** 72–80

Powles RL, Russell J, Lister TA *et al* (1977) Immunotherapy for AML: analysis of a controlled clinical study 2+ years after entry of the last patient. *British Journal of Cancer* **35** 265

Proby C, Storey A, McGregor J and Leigh I (1996) Does human papillomavirus infection play a role in non-melanoma skin cancer? *Papillomavirus Report* **7** 53–60

Pugh RCB (1973) The pathology of cancer of the bladder: an editorial overview. *Cancer* **32** 1267–1274

Read B, French P and Singer A (1978) Sperm basic proteins in cervical carcinogenesis: correlation with socioeconomic class. *Lancet* **ii** 60–64

Richardson A and Lyon J (1981) The effect of condom use in squamous cell cervical intra-epithelial neoplasia. *American Journal of Obstetrics and Gynaecology* **140** 909–913

Rotola A, Monini P, Di Luca D *et al* (1992) Presence and physical state of HPV DNA in prostate and urinary-tract tissues. *International Journal of Cancer* **52** 359–65

Rous P and Beard J (1935) The progression to carcinoma of virus-induced rabbit papillomas

(Shope). *Journal of Experimental Medicine* **62** 523–548

Rous P and Kidd J (1936) The carcinogenic effect of a virus upon tarred skin. *Science* **83** 468–469

Rovere GQD, Oliver RTD, McCance DJ and Castro JE (1988) Development of bladder tumour containing HPV type 11 DNA after renal transplantation. *British Journal of Urology* **62** 36–38

Saltzstein DR, Orihuela E, Kocurek JN *et al* (1993) Failure of the polymerase chain reaction (PCR) to detect human papilloma virus (HPV) in transitional cell carcinoma of the bladder. *Anticancer Research* **13** 423–425

Sano T, Sakurai S, Fukuda T and Nakajima T (1995) Unsuccessful effort to detect human papillomavirus DNA in urinary bladder cancers by the polymerase chain reaction and in situ hybridization. *Pathology International* **45** 506–512

Schulz T, Boshoff C and Weiss R (1996) HIV infection and neoplasia. *Lancet* **348** 589–591

Shamanin V, zur Hausen H, Lavergne D *et al* (1996) Human papillomavirus infections in non-melanoma skin cancers from renal transplant recipients and nonimmunosuppressed patients. *Journal of the National Cancer Institute* **88** 802–811

Shibutani YF, Schoenberg MP, Carpiniello VL and Malloy TR (1992) Human papillomavirus associated with bladder cancer. *Urology* **40** 15–17

Shindoh M, Chiba I, Yasuda M *et al* (1995) Detection of human papillomavirus DNA sequences in oral squamous cell carcinomas and their relation to p53 and proliferating cell nuclear antigen expression. *Cancer* **76** 1513–1521

Siegsmund M, Wayss K and Amtmann E (1991) Activation of latent papillomavirus genomes by chronic mechanical irritation. *Journal of General Virology* **72** 2787–2789

Sinclair AL, Nouri AME, Oliver RTD, Sexton C and Dalgleish AG (1993) Bladder and prostate cancer screening for human papillomavirus by polymerase chain reaction: conflicting results using different annealing temperatures. *British Journal of Biomedical Science* **50** 350–354

Straight SW, Herman B and McCance DJ (1995) The E5 oncoprotein of human papillomavirus type 16 inhibits the acidification of endosomes in human keratinocytes. *Journal of Virology* **69** 3185–3192

Vogelstein B, Fearon E, Kern S *et al* (1989) Allelotype of colorectal carcinomas. *Science* **244** 207–211

Vousden K (1994) Mechanisms of transformation by HPV, In: Stern P and Stanley M (eds). *Human Papillomaviruses and Cervical Cancer* pp 92–115, Oxford University Press, Oxford

Wiener JS, Liu ET and Walther PJ (1992) Oncogenic human papillomavirus type 16 is associated with squamous cell cancer of the male urethra. *Cancer Research* **52** 5018–5023

Wilson RW, Chenggis ML and Unger ER (1990) Longitudinal study of human papillomavirus infection of the female urogenital tract by in situ hybridization. *Archives of Pathology and Laboratory Medicine* **114** 155–159

Yeudall WA and Campo MS (1991) Human papillomavirus DNA in biopsies of oral tissues. *Journal of General Virology* **72** 173–176

Young L, Bevan I, Johnson M *et al* (1989) The polymerase chain reaction: a new epidemiological tool for investigating cervical human papillomavirus infection. *British Medical Journal* **298** 14–18

Zunzunegui MV, King MC, Coria CF and Charlet J (1986) Male influences on cervical cancer risk. *American Journal of Epidemiology* **123** 302–307

zur Hausen H (1991) Human papillomaviruses in the pathogenesis of anogenital cancer. *Virology* **184** 9–13

zur Hausen H (1994) Molecular pathogenesis of cancer of the cervix and its causation by specific human papillomavirus types. *Current Topics in Microbiology and Immunology* **186** 131–156

The authors are responsible for the accuracy of the references.

Molecular Genetics of Bladder Cancer: Pathways of Development and Progression

MARGARET A. KNOWLES*

*Molecular Genetics Laboratory, Marie Curie Research Institute,
The Chart, Oxted, Surrey RH8 0TL*

Introduction
**Pathogenesis of transitional cell carcinoma of the bladder: two major
    progression pathways?**
Genetic susceptibility to bladder cancer
Somatic alterations in transitional cell carcinoma
    Oncogene activation
        RAS *gene mutation*
        ERBB2 *amplification and overexpression*
        Amplification of genes at 11q13
    Chromosomal deletions, allelic loss and tumour suppressor genes
        CDKN2 *and chromosome 9*
        TP53 *and 17p*
        RB *and 13q*
    Other genomic regions with loss of heterozygosity
    DNA repair defects
Genetic alterations in carcinoma in situ
Genetic alterations in schistosomiasis associated bladder cancer
A molecular genetic progression model for transitional cell carcinoma
Summary and future directions

INTRODUCTION

Tumour development and progression involves the accumulation of multiple heritable cellular alterations over a long period of time. Sequential selection and expansion of altered clones at each stage of the process can lead ultimately to the evolution of a highly anaplastic and metastatic phenotype. Work on many tumour types, including bladder cancer, indicates that the events that contribute to this process can be genetic (mutation) or epigenetic (eg DNA methylation) but invariably each change alters the function of a gene with a critical role in cell proliferation or differentiation.

*Present address: ICRF Cancer Medicine Research Unit, St James's University Hospital, Beckett Street, Leeds LS9 7TF.

Cancer Surveys Volume 31: *Bladder Cancer*
© 1998 Imperial Cancer Research Fund. 0-87969-529-3/98. $5.00 + .00

Epidemiological evidence suggests that, as for most solid tumours, six to eight events may be required for the development of a bladder tumour (Cook *et al*, 1969). During the past decade, rapid advances in molecular genetic technology have led to the identification of a profusion of genetic alterations in human cancer and the catalogue of known genetic alterations in bladder cancer is now substantial. This rapid expansion of knowledge has been fuelled by the prediction that an understanding of the genetics of the disease will provide both insight into the diverse clinical phenotypes of bladder tumours and tools that can be applied to aid in diagnosis and prediction of prognosis and in the design of novel therapies.

Now that many key genes have been identified, we are ready to embark on the more exciting and inevitably more exacting task of applying this knowledge to the benefit of patients with bladder cancer. This chapter reviews the nature of the genetic alterations found in carcinoma of the bladder and their association with clinical phenotype and outlines some current hypotheses on the timing of events, their relevance to disease progression and possible clinical applications.

PATHOGENESIS OF TRANSITIONAL CELL CARCINOMA OF THE BLADDER: TWO MAJOR PROGRESSION PATHWAYS?

At presentation, approximately 80% of transitional cell carcinomas (TCC) of the bladder are superficial papillary lesions (T_a/T_1), the majority of which will show no propensity to invade despite the common development of recurrences at the same or different sites in the bladder over a period of many years. For most of the 20% of tumours which are muscle invasive $(\geq T_2)$ or metastatic (N+, M+) at the time of presentation, there is apparently no superficial papillary precursor lesion and these tumours may be rapidly fatal (Koss, 1975). An overwhelming weight of evidence (histopathological, clinical, molecular) suggests that these different modes of presentation and contrasting clinical outcome indicate the existence of two distinct disease processes and the genetic evidence for this will be discussed in later sections.

The natural history of these two proposed disease entities is not absolutely clear, due to several confounding features. One of these is the common finding of several lesions simultaneously in the same bladder, the developmental relationship between which is unknown. Similarly, new or recurrent tumours may develop at the same or different sites in the bladder over the course of the disease. The difficulty in interpreting the evolution of such tumours contrasts with the situation in other tissues where a single primary tumour is the rule and where the presence, for example, of a focus of overt carcinoma within a benign lesion, is highly suggestive of the sequence of biological events. For bladder cancer, it may be predicted that the use of genetic markers may clarify the situation, and indeed this has been and continues to be the case.

GENETIC SUSCEPTIBILITY TO BLADDER CANCER

In several human cancers, for example breast, prostate, testis, there is a clear familial genetic component. This is far less clear for cancer of the bladder, but there is some evidence for an increased risk in persons with a family history of bladder cancer. Kantor *et al* (1985) reported on a population based study of 2982 bladder cancer patients and 5782 controls in the United States to assess the role of environmental risk factors and history of urinary tract cancer in first degree relatives. An elevation of risk was found in patients with a family history (relative risk 1.45) and this was significantly higher in heavy smokers (relative risk 10.7 among those who smoked ≥3 packs per day).

This higher risk in smokers suggests that there may be an interaction between smoking and familial predisposition. A possible mechanism for this may be genetic polymorphism in enzymes involved in metabolism of the carcinogens present in cigarette smoke. Interindividual variability in the metabolism of arylamines by the *N*-acetyltransferases (NAT1 and NAT2) has been identified and a series of mutant alleles of NAT2 have been characterized that give rise to so called "slow" and "fast" acetylator phenotypes. Several studies link the "slow" acetylator phenotype that is present in 50% of individuals to a higher risk of bladder cancer (Cartwright *et al*, 1982; Risch *et al*, 1995). Similarly, inheritance of glutathione S-transferase M1(*GSTM1*) deficiency, which is determined by complete deletion of the gene, has been shown to confer a higher risk of bladder cancer (Bell *et al*, 1993; Brockmoller *et al*, 1995). It is possible that other inherited variations in the ability to activate or detoxify other types of carcinogen may also have considerable impact.

Evidence for familial clustering is less clear cut and to date no extended pedigrees with increased risk of bladder cancer have been reported. However, there are reports of small family clusters with several cases in first degree relatives, some diagnosed in individuals less than 40 years old and with no obvious history of occupational exposure or smoking (eg McCullough *et al*, 1975; Lynch *et al*, 1979, 1987). These familial clusters of bladder carcinoma in which the apparent risk of disease is far greater than that associated with inherited variation in metabolic capacity may represent inheritance of a mutated allele of a gene involved in control of cell proliferation or differentiation, as is the case in several familial cancer syndromes. Since it is predicted that more than six genetic events are required for bladder cancer development, the inheritance of one mutant allele via the germline would not be expected to have as obvious an effect on tumour incidence as in tumour types where fewer genetic events are required. Cases would occur relatively late in life and, unless careful attention was paid to family history, clusters involving several generations might not be recognized. It is quite possible therefore that bladder cancer may have a much stronger familial component than has previously been recognized. This emphasizes the need for meticulous documentation of both environmental exposure and family history in all cases. Examination of families for evidence for genetic linkage could now be attempted. The identification of many specific genetic alterations in bladder cancer provides a useful starting point for linkage studies and since polymerase chain reaction based analysis can be carried out on normal and tumour DNA extracted from archival material, access to family clusters described in the past would be possible.

SOMATIC ALTERATIONS IN TRANSITIONAL CELL CARCINOMA

Since no clear familial predisposition to carcinoma of the bladder has been identified, all genetic events identified to date are considered to have occurred somatically. Alterations to both proto-oncogenes and tumour suppressor genes have been found.

Cytogenetic findings of several non-random alterations in bladder cancer specimens gave an early indication of regions of the genome likely to be involved. These include monosomy 9, i(5p), monosomy 8 or 8p-, 11p-, 21q- and trisomy 7. Cytogenetic findings have been reviewed in detail recently (Sandberg and Berger, 1994) and will not be discussed here. Many of the cytogenetic deletions described have been confirmed by molecular assays.

Oncogene Activation

Several proto-oncogenes are implicated in the development of TCC. However, due to the difficulties inherent in screening for novel oncogenes, in recent years most attention has focused on the identification of tumour suppressor genes. One approach that has proved useful in identifying genomic regions that show gross amplification in tumour tissues is the technique of comparative genomic hybridization and this was applied recently to a series of bladder tumours (Kallioniemi *et al*, 1995). Gains of DNA sequences were found in more than 10% of tumours at 8q21, 13q21-34, 1q31, 3q24-26 and 1p22. None of these regions contains known oncogenes.

RAS *Gene Mutation*

There has been controversy regarding the frequency of *RAS* gene mutation in bladder cancer. Initial studies using functional assays estimated that 7–16% of bladder tumours contained a *RAS* oncogene (Fujita *et al*, 1985; Malone *et al*, 1985). More recent results using molecular genetic techniques have yielded a much wider range of results. Two recent studies of *HRAS*, both of which were well controlled and used robust techniques, detected G→T mutations at codon 12 (Gly→Val) in 26 of 62 (42%) T_a/T_1 tumours (Ooi *et al*, 1994) and exon 1 mutations in 44% of urine sediments from patients at the time of presentation with bladder cancer (Fitzgerald *et al*, 1995) respectively. In the study of Ooi *et al* (1994), no significant association was found between *RAS* mutation and tumour recurrence or progression. Since it is clear from transfection experiments into bladder carcinoma cell lines (Theodorescu *et al*, 1991) and non-tumorigenic human urothelial cells at different stages during in vitro progression (Pratt *et al*, 1992) that mutated *HRAS* has profound effects on urothelial cell phenotype, further exploration of the timing, prevalence and clinical implications of mutation during tumour progression in vivo is merited.

ERBB2 *Amplification and Overexpression*

The proto-oncogene *ERBB2* is amplified and/or overexpressed in many epithelial cancers including bladder cancer. Gross amplification of the gene is found in some tumours, predominantly high grade, high stage lesions (Zhau *et al*, 1990; Coombs *et al*, 1991). Expression of the protein is confined to the luminal surface of mature superficial urothelial cells in the normal bladder. In tumours, overexpression can be detected by immunohistochemistry in all tumours with gene amplification and in many tumours without. This has been confirmed by several independent studies (eg Coombs *et al*, 1991; Sato *et al*, 1992; Sauter *et al*, 1993; Mellon *et al*, 1996). It appears that overexpression may have some use as a prognostic indicator. Sato *et al* (1992) reported a clear association of overexpression with poor clinical outcome and a recent study of 236 tumours from 89 patients by Underwood *et al* (1995) found that in multivariate analysis, ERBB2 protein overexpression and gene amplification had predictive value for death from bladder cancer. However, tumour grade and stage remained the most important prognostic variables.

Amplification of Genes at 11q13

Approximately 20% of bladder tumours show amplification of sequences at 11q13 (Proctor *et al*, 1991). A likely target of these amplifications is the *CCND1* (cyclin D1) gene, which is involved in control of progression from the G_1 to S phases of the cell cycle. There is evidence of overexpression of the gene in tumours with amplification (Bringuier *et al*, 1994). Another possible target gene in this region is *EMS1*, which is co-amplified in most tumours with 11q13 amplification and is also overexpressed (Bringuier *et al*, 1996). There is no apparent association between tumour grade and/or stage or clinical outcome and gene amplification in this region.

Chromosomal Deletions, Allelic Loss and Tumour Suppressor Genes

CDKN2 *and Chromosome 9*

Alterations to chromosome 9 are the most frequent cytogenetic and molecular genetic findings in bladder tumours of all grades and stages (Tsai *et al*, 1990; Cairns *et al*, 1993a). Several studies of large numbers of tumours have reported loss of heterozygosity (LOH) at all informative loci on chromosome 9 in the vast majority of cases, indicating that the most common event involving chromosome 9 is loss of an entire copy. This almost certainly reflects the presence on both arms of the chromosome of tumour suppressor genes that participate in bladder cancer development. However, a few tumours show deletions that involve only part of the chromosome and this has allowed mapping of putative critical regions within which tumour suppressor genes are predicted to lie.

Detailed mapping of partial deletions of 9p has identified a region close to the interferon gene cluster at 9p21 (Cairns *et al*, 1994; Devlin *et al*, 1994). Within this common region of deletion are p16 (*CDKN2/INK4A/MTS1*) and p15 (*INK4B/MTS2*), both negative cell cycle regulators. *CDKN2* is deleted or mutated at high frequency in many tumour types (Kamb *et al*, 1994; Nobori *et al*, 1994) and has been shown to represent one of the familial melanoma loci (Hussussian *et al*, 1994). The region including *CDKN2* and *INK4B* is homozygously deleted in a large proportion of bladder carcinoma cell lines (Kamb *et al*, 1994; Spruck *et al*, 1994a) and bladder tumours in vivo (Cairns *et al*, 1995; Orlow *et al*, 1995; Williamson *et al*, 1995). Rare examples of retention of *CDKN2* with deletion of *INK4B* and retention of *INK4B* with deletion of *CDKN2* have been described (Orlow *et al*, 1995; Williamson *et al*, 1995), implicating both genes in bladder cancer development. Sequence analysis of *CDKN2* has revealed few mutations in bladder tumours (Spruck *et al*, 1994a; Gruis *et al*, 1995; Williamson *et al*, 1995) and it appears that homozygous deletion is the major genetic mechanism of inactivation. There is the suggestion from one study that the frequency of deletion is higher in low stage papillary tumours (Orlow *et al*, 1995). Other studies, however, show no obvious association with either tumour grade or stage.

In addition to frequent inactivation by homozygous deletion, loss of one allele and silencing by methylation of the retained allele represents an alternative mechanism for *CDKN2* inactivation (Gonzalez-Zulueta *et al*, 1995a). Methylation associated silencing of *INK4B* was not found in the 18 uncultured bladder tumours studied by these authors. The proportions of tumours with 9p LOH that show homozygous deletion or methylation of *CDKN2* have not yet been estimated. It is possible that some tumours with no detectable deletion have methylation based silencing of both alleles.

Confirmation of the role of *CDKN2* in bladder tumour development has come from gene replacement studies (Wu *et al*, 1996). Introduction of a *CDKN2* cDNA under control of the cytomegalovirus promoter into two bladder carcinoma cell lines that lack wild type *CDKN2*, led to a tenfold reduction in the number of stable transfectant colonies obtained, compared with vector alone. All clones obtained showed rearrangement of the introduced *CDKN2* sequence, indicating a growth inhibitory effect of the wild type sequence. Similarly, introduction of a normal human chromosome 9 by microcell mediated chromosome transfer yielded a majority of clones in which deletion of the

9p21 region on the introduced chromosome had occurred. To date, *INK4B* alone has not been reintroduced into bladder carcinoma cells.

Since *CDKN2* is known to be involved in a pathway that ultimately regulates the retinoblastoma susceptibility gene *(RB)* function, it will be interesting to ask whether inactivations of these two genes are independent events in bladder cancer since in other tumour types (eg lung cancer) inactivation of *CDKN2* and *RB* appear to be mutually exclusive (Shapiro *et al*, 1995). To date a comprehensive study has not been reported, but it has been shown that in some instances where the *RB* gene is known to be defective, *CDKN2* is clearly intact and protein levels are upregulated (Yeager *et al*, 1995). Since TP53 is not directly involved in this pathway, *TP53* mutation might not be expected to be related to *CDKN2* or *RB* inactivation, and indeed there is evidence that mutation of *TP53* is independent of *CDKN2* alterations in bladder cancer (Gruis *et al*, 1995).

Fine mapping of the putative tumour suppressor genes on 9q has proved extremely difficult as subchromosomal deletions involving 9q only are rarer than those of 9p and the deleted region in those cases that have been identified is usually large. Seven large studies during the past 4 years involving >700 tumours (Cairns *et al*, 1993b; Miyao *et al*, 1993; Ruppert *et al*, 1993; Keen and Knowles, 1994; Habuchi *et al*, 1995, 1997; Simoneau *et al*, 1996) have identified only 48 cases with partial deletion of 9q (6.7%). Three common regions of deletion have been defined: a very large centromeric region encompassing the Gorlin syndrome gene *(PTC)*, a region at 9q34 between D9S61 and D9S66 (estimated as 13–14 cM) and a third region at 9q32-33 close to D9S195. The latter region (Habuchi *et al*, 1997) is the most precisely mapped and five tumours with very small interstitial deletions have been described. Interestingly, all of these were low grade, low stage tumours. Identification of the target gene within this region which is <840 kb should follow shortly. Mutation analyses (Simoneau *et al*, 1996; Shaw ME and Knowles MA, unpublished) indicate that the target gene within the more centromeric 9q region is not *PTC*. At 9q34, the critical region is coincident with that for the tuberous sclerosis 1 locus *(TSC1)*, which has been shown to behave as a tumour suppressor gene (Carbonara *et al*, 1994; Green *et al*, 1994) and this gene, now identified (van Stegtenhorst *et al*, 1997), is a good candidate for the bladder tumour suppressor in the region.

Several studies have found no association between chromosome 9 LOH and bladder tumour grade or stage. More than 50% of tumours studied have shown LOH on 9q (Cairns *et al*, 1993a). Figure 1 illustrates the proportions of tumours that showed LOH on 9p and 9q in a series of 95 tumours we studied (Keen and Knowles, 1994). In the majority of cases, where the entire chromosome shows LOH, the number of genes inactivated is unknown. Thus, until each relevant tumour suppressor gene on chromosome 9 has been identified it will not be possible to make an objective assessment of any clinical associations.

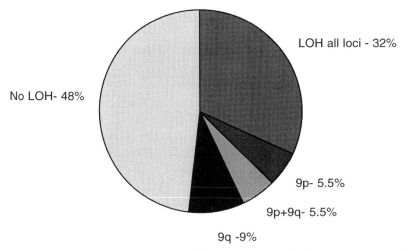

Fig. 1. Location of chromosome 9 deletions in transitional cell carcinoma of the bladder. 9p and 9q indicate discrete deletions on each chromosome arm

TP53 and 17p

Allele loss on chromosome 17p is frequent in TCC (Olumi *et al*, 1990; Tsai *et al*, 1990; Habuchi *et al*, 1993a; Knowles *et al*, 1994) and is most frequent in tumours of high grade and stage. In the majority of cases, 17p LOH is associated with mutation of the *TP53* gene on the retained allele (Sidransky *et al*, 1991; Habuchi *et al*, 1993b; Williamson *et al*, 1994). In the many studies that have examined *TP53* mutations in bladder tumours, mutations have been found in most tumours with 17p LOH, but as in other types of tumour there is also some evidence for LOH in a region telomeric to *TP53* on 17p. There is a clear association of *TP53* mutation with tumour grade and stage. For example, Fujimoto *et al* (1992) found mutations in 6 of 12 invasive tumours studied but only 1 of 13 superficial tumours.

Because bladder cancer is a smoking related cancer, particular attention has been paid to the mutation spectrum of *TP53* in these tumours. Comparison of bladder cancers from smokers and non-smokers has revealed the presence of multiple or tandem mutations and an excess of A:T→G:C transitions in the tumours of current smokers (Spruck *et al*, 1993). When compared with lung cancer (smoking related) and colorectal carcinoma (non-smoking related), bladder cancer has a distinct *TP53* mutation spectrum (Sidransky *et al*, 1991; Habuchi *et al*, 1993b; Spruck *et al*, 1993). In particular, a significantly higher frequency of G:C→C:G transversions has been found in bladder cancer. It has been suggested that such mutations may be induced by oxygen free radicals present in cigarette smoke. The known bladder carcinogen 4-aminobiphenyl, also present in cigarette smoke, induces predominantly G:C→T:A and A:T→T:A mutations, which have not been found at high frequency.

The association of *TP53* mutation with high tumour grade and stage suggests that *TP53* status may have prognostic significance. Mutant TP53 protein commonly exhibits an extended half life and mutant protein accumulates in the nucleus. This can be detected by immunohistochemistry, whereas wild type TP53 in the absence of mutant protein is not detectable. Several studies have concluded that accumulation of the TP53 protein is an independent prognostic marker in bladder cancer (Lipponen, 1993; Sarkis *et al*, 1993a,b; Soini *et al*, 1993; Cordon-Cardo *et al*, 1994; Esrig *et al*, 1994). In the study of Esrig *et al* (1994) nuclear TP53 reactivity was related to time to tumour recurrence and overall survival in 243 patients treated with radical cystectomy. A significant association of nuclear TP53 with increased risk of recurrence and overall survival was found for T_1, T_2 and T_{3a} tumours. Similarly, in patients with carcinoma in situ, T_a or T_1 papillary tumours that were treated by local resection or intravesical bacille Calmette-Guérin therapy, disease progression (muscle invasion/ metastasis/death) was associated with TP53 immunoreactivity (Sarkis *et al*, 1993a,b, 1994).

The finding that TP53 altered cells are less able to undergo apoptosis (Lowe *et al*, 1993) led to the view that TP53 altered tumours are likely to be more resistant to chemotherapy. Since prediction of the likely response of tumours to chemotherapy could have profound implications in the selection of patients who would benefit from such treatment, the response to chemotherapy of bladder tumours with known TP53 status was recently examined (Cote *et al*, 1997). In a group of patients with locally invasive bladder cancer in whom TP53 status had shown a clear association with increased risk of tumour progression, it was found that of those who received chemotherapy after cystectomy, the patients with altered TP53 status showed a lower relative risk of tumour recurrence or death. These results are consistent with the results of a recent study by Waldman *et al* (1996) that showed that cells with mutated TP53 show uncoupling of S phase and mitosis and are highly susceptible to radiation or doxorubicin induced apoptosis. If confirmed, these results indicate that while TP53 mutation confirms a higher risk in untreated patients, TP53 altered tumours may benefit most from chemotherapy.

While nuclear TP53 staining appears to be predictive of a high risk of tumour progression, absence of TP53 staining does not, however, guarantee a low risk. This may reflect the presence in some tumours of TP53 mutations such as protein truncations that do not lead to accumulation of high protein levels. Alternatively, other factors may contribute to tumour progression in these cases. Some may be attributed to *RB* mutations (see below), but some may have alterations to other genes involved in the same signalling pathway as TP53. Alterations to the *MDM2* gene, which encodes a TP53 binding protein that can abrogate normal TP53 function, have been identified in some tumours (Habuchi *et al*, 1994). Amplification of *MDM2* was found in two high grade invasive tumours without TP53 mutation (Habuchi *et al*, 1994). Using immunohistochemistry, Lianes *et al* (1994) found gene amplification in only a single tumour but overexpression of MDM2 protein in a large proportion of tumours (26 of 87) and this was associated with TP53 overexpression and found predominantly in low grade, low stage tumours. The significance of this finding is not yet clear. More recently, alternatively spliced *MDM2* transcripts that show loss of TP53 binding ability have been identified in several tumour samples including bladder (Sigalas *et al*, 1996). Only 1 of 16 superficial (T_a/T_1) tumours showed evidence of alternatively spliced transcripts compared with 4 of 7 muscle invasive tumours. The altered transcripts identified were shown to have transforming activity in NIH 3T3 cells in vitro despite loss of the TP53 binding domain. This indicates that *MDM2* may have transforming activity which is TP53 independent. Other genes involved in potential TP53 related pathways have not yet been studied in bladder cancer.

RB and 13q

The retinoblastoma susceptibility gene (*RB*) on chromosome 13q is implicated in the development of muscle invasive bladder cancer. LOH at the *RB* locus is present in a significant number of bladder tumours (Cairns *et al*, 1991; Ishikawa *et al*, 1991) and this shows a striking association with muscle invasion (Cairns *et al*, 1991). RNA-single stranded conformation polymorphism (SSCP) and sequencing has identified mutations in the retained allele in bladder tumours with LOH (Miyamoto *et al*, 1995). The protein product can be clearly demonstrated in normal cells by immunohistochemistry and loss of RB protein expression correlates with LOH at the *RB* locus (Xu *et al*, 1993). Two studies have demonstrated a clear association of loss of RB expression with more aggressive clinical behaviour of tumours indicating that *RB* inactivation may be an important prognostic marker (Cordon-Cardo *et al*, 1992; Logothetis *et al*, 1992). In a study of 48 tumours, Cordon-Cardo *et al* (1992) found altered RB protein expression in 14 tumours and all but one of these were muscle invasive. Survival was significantly decreased in RB altered cases (p<0.001). Similarly, Logothetis *et al* (1992) found altered RB expression in 16 of 43 locally invasive tumours examined and these showed a significantly decreased tumour free survival rate. Therefore, as for TP53, inactivation of *RB* appears to be a useful negative prognostic indicator in muscle invasive bladder cancer. As yet, a large study of superficial tumours with complete clinical follow up has not been reported. However, it has recently been reported that in a group of 28 T_a and 31 T_1 tumours there was a strong association of undetectable RB expression with disease progression (p=0.006) (Cordon-Cardo *et al*, 1997). In this study, TP53 positivity was also associated with disease progression (p=0.001) and, most interestingly, alterations to both genes were observed in 9 cases (of 11 with undetectable RB). This significant association between the two alterations has not been identified before and showed an even more marked association with progression (p=0.00005). This suggests that TP53 and RB alterations may have a cooperative effect as has been suggested by the phenotype of mice heterozygous for mutations in both genes (Williams *et al*, 1994). Prospective clinical studies using large, well characterized groups of patients are now needed.

Other Genomic Regions with Loss of Heterozygosity

An allelotype analysis of 83 bladder tumours (Knowles *et al*, 1994) identified LOH not only in the region of known tumour suppressor genes including 17p (TP53), 13q (*RB*) and 9p (*CDKN2*), but in several other regions of the genome including 4p, 8p, 9q and 11p. LOH has also been reported on chromosome arms 18q (Brewster *et al*, 1994), 3p (Presti *et al*, 1991) and 14q (Chang *et al*, 1995). The target tumour suppressor genes of these deletions have not yet been identified. A representation of combined data from several studies of LOH in TCC is shown in Fig. 2. The data depicted are from Knowles *et al* (1994) for all chromosome arms except 3p, 4q, 14q and 18q where data are from other studies (Presti *et al*, 1991; Brewster *et al*, 1994; Chang *et al*, 1995; Polascik *et al*, 1995), which showed higher frequencies of LOH, presumably due to selection of polymorphic markers closer to critical regions of deletion.

Three regions of deletion have been mapped on chromosome 4, one at 4p16.3 (Elder *et al*, 1994; Bell *et al*, 1996), one at 4p15 and one on 4q (Polascik *et al*, 1995). There is also evidence for a region of deletion close to the centromere but this has not been mapped in detail (Elder *et al*, 1994). A candidate gene *SH3BP2* (homologue of the mouse Sh3bp2 gene, a known SH3 domain binding protein) has been identified within the 40 kb critical region at 4p16.3

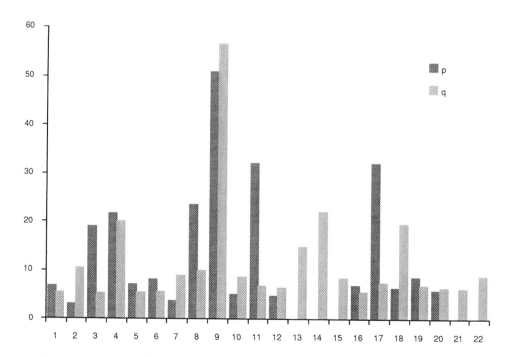

Fig. 2. Allelotype of transitional cell carcinoma. Each bar represents the percentage of tumours from informative patients that showed LOH. Data from Knowles *et al* (1994), Presti *et al* (1991), Brewster *et al* (1994), Polascik *et al* (1995) and Chang *et al* (1995)—see text

but to date no tumour specific inactivating mutations have been identified (Bell *et al*, 1997). Deletions in this telomeric region are found in ~22% of tumours and show no association with tumour grade or stage. LOH in the more proximal region on 4p was found in 29% of tumours and on 4q in 24% and LOH in both regions showed a significant association with advanced grade and stage (Polascik *et al*, 1995).

Deletion of markers on chromosome 8p is found in ~22% of bladder cancers and this shows a strong association with tumour grade and stage (Knowles *et al*, 1993). A complex pattern of deletions has been found. Many deletions encompass a region at 8p21 that is deleted in other cancers including prostate, colorectal and hepatocellular carcinomas (Bergerheim *et al*, 1991; Emi *et al*, 1993; Fujiwara *et al*, 1993). In addition, two or possibly three more proximal regions are implicated by LOH analysis (Takle and Knowles, 1996). Several candidate genes on 8p including *NAT1*, *NAT2*, *POLB*, and *PPP2CB* have either been excluded from the deleted regions or have shown no mutations by SSCP or sequence analysis in bladder tumours (Eydmann and Knowles, 1997; Shaw ME, Knowles MA and Luscombe M, unpublished). Since 53% of muscle invasive TCCs show LOH on 8p, identification of the target gene(s) represents an important step in understanding the biology of bladder cancer progression.

LOH of markers on 11p was the earliest deletion reported in bladder cancer (Fearon *et al*, 1985). LOH of 11p is found in ~40% of all bladder tumours (Tsai *et al*, 1990; Presti *et al*, 1991; Dalbagni *et al*, 1993; Habuchi *et al*, 1993a; Knowles *et al*, 1994). Although there is some suggestion that these deletions are more frequent in tumours of high grade, the association is not striking. A study using fluorescence in situ hybridization to detect chromosome 11 centromere and both p and q arms has confirmed loss of an entire copy of chromosome 11 or underrepresentation of 11p in many non-diploid TCCs (Voorter *et al*, 1996). The frequency of monosomy or 11p loss in this study was 13 of 16 (81%) in non-diploid tumours. Since this type of analysis is less likely to be affected by normal tissue contamination of the tumour sample, it appears that involvement of chromosome 11 deletion may be more frequent than indicated from LOH analyses. Detailed deletion mapping of chromosome 11 has shown that the critical region is at 11p15. A region of deletion on 11q between 11q13 and 11q23 was also identified (Shaw and Knowles, 1995). The 11p region does not include *HRAS* or *WT1* and to date no candidate genes have been identified on either 11p or 11q.

LOH of 3p and 18q is found in ~30% of tumours and in both cases is associated with high tumour grade and stage (Presti *et al*, 1991; Brewster *et al*, 1994). Three critical regions of 3p have been implicated in other tumour types but as yet no detailed mapping in bladder cancer has been carried out, though a region at 3p12-p14.2 has been implicated from studies of in vitro transformation of human urothelial cells (Klingelhutz *et al*, 1991). On 18q, the common region of deletion is at 18q21.3-qter and includes the *DCC* locus. LOH on 14q has been reported in 25% of bladder tumours and two small common regions of deletion at 14q12 (2 cM) and 14q32.1-32.2 (3 cM) have been mapped (Chang *et al*, 1995). LOH in this study was more common in invasive tumours.

It is of interest that many of the regions of deletion mapped by LOH analysis have also been identified as regions of loss by comparative genomic hybridization (Kallioniemi *et al*, 1995). These include 11p, 11q, 8p, 9, 17p, 18q and 3p. In addition, losses of 2q, 10q and 16 were found. No known tumour suppressor genes are mapped within any of these regions except *PTEN* at 10q23.

DNA Repair Defects

Hereditary non-polyposis colorectal cancer has been causally linked to mutations in one of a series of mismatch repair genes (*MSH2, MLH1, PMS1, PMS2*), defects that generate genetic instability which is characterized by the generation of multiple length variations in microsatellites (Perucho, 1997). Such a phenotype of microsatellite instability has been identified in several types of sporadic cancer including bladder cancer. The frequency of generalized instability giving rise to alterations at multiple loci is relatively low, only 3 of 200 tumours examined by Gonzalez-Zulueta *et al* (1993) showing multiple alterations. All of these tumours were T_a or T_1 tumours. Mutation analysis of the mismatch repair genes that may be responsible for such alterations has not been carried out.

Clonal alterations affecting at least one microsatellite marker are more common and have been tested as a means to screen urine samples from patients presenting with symptoms suggestive of bladder cancer (Mao *et al*, 1996). In such cases, it is likely that the alterations occurred spontaneously and appear clonal due to the concomitant acquisition of some other alteration that confers a selective advantage. Microsatellite markers shown in a preliminary study to undergo frequent alteration and markers that show frequent LOH in bladder cancer were studied in 25 symptomatic cases and 5 controls. Nineteen of 20 (95%) patients in whom bladder cancer was diagnosed were detected by this analysis, compared with a detection rate of 50% using routine cytology.

GENETIC ALTERATIONS IN CARCINOMA IN SITU

Carcinoma in situ (CIS) is by definition a high grade lesion in which normal thickness urothelium (five to seven cell layers) shows severe dysplasia in the absence of invasion. CIS as the sole abnormality in the bladder is a high risk lesion with invasive disease developing in 60% of cases within 5 years (Koss 1979; Lamm, 1992). Because of the high probability of progression compared with superficial papillary tumours, CIS has long been proposed to be a precursor lesion for flat invasive bladder tumours. The presence of CIS may be suspected at surgery but since histological confirmation is required, fresh tissue specimens are not generally available. Thus molecular analysis of CIS is difficult and relies on microdissection of small areas from histological sections. Nevertheless, there is a significant amount of molecular genetic information.

Rosin *et al* (1995) carried out a partial allelotyping of 31 archival cases of CIS. LOH analysis was carried out on 13 chromosome arms previously implicated in TCC (3p, 4p, 4q, 5q, 8p, 9p, 9q, 11p, 11q, 13q, 14q, 17p and 18q). A comparison of the frequency of LOH on these chromosome arms compared with that found in TCC is shown in Fig. 3. A significantly higher frequency of LOH on 8p, 14q and 17p was found than in TCC specimens unselected for grade and stage. All these changes are found much more commonly in high grade, high stage TCC and their presence in CIS is compatible with this being a high grade lesion and a precursor for these more aggressive tumours. Interestingly, 18q LOH was not found at significantly higher frequency (29%) than in unselected TCCs (~30%).

Spruck *et al* (1994b) examined 21 examples of CIS and 5 dysplasias (classified as moderate or severe) for LOH of 9q and for *TP53* mutation; 15 of 23 of these contained a *TP53* mutation, a frequency similar to that expected in high grade invasive TCC. In contrast, LOH of chromosome 9 was found in only 3 of 24 cases. This frequency (12%) is significantly different from that seen in either papillary or flat invasive bladder tumours, all of which show >50% LOH. These findings for *TP53* involvement in CIS have been confirmed by Wagner *et al*

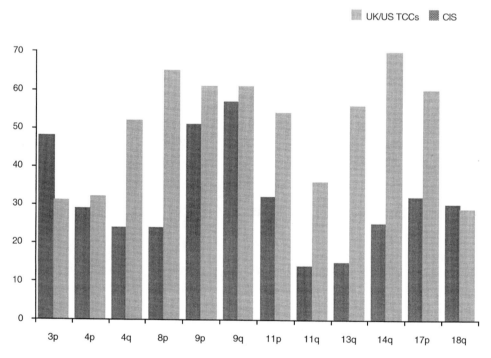

Fig. 3. Comparison of the frequency of LOH on selected chromosome arms in CIS (data from Rosin *et al*, 1995) and TCC (data from Presti *et al*, 1991; Knowles *et al*, 1993; Brewster *et al*, 1994; Chang *et al*, 1995; Polascik *et al*, 1995)

(1995) who studied expression of TP53 and ERBB2 by immunohistochemistry in 20 cases of CIS and compared them with normal and mildly dysplastic urothelium. TP53 and ERBB2 positivity were associated with CIS (7 of 20 and 12 of 20 respectively) and all 7 cases with TP53 overexpression also showed diffuse overexpression of ERBB2. Again these findings closely resemble what is found in high grade invasive TCC.

GENETIC ALTERATIONS IN SCHISTOSOMIASIS ASSOCIATED BLADDER CANCER

Schistosomiasis (bilharzia) is a parasitic disease, endemic in 75 countries and affecting more than 200 million people world wide (WHO, 1985). In Egypt, where it is hyperendemic, more than 20% of the population are infected and there are high rates of morbidity and mortality. One of the consequences of infection with *Schistosoma haematobium* is a marked increase in the incidence of carcinoma of the bladder (IARC, 1994). In Egypt for example, bladder cancer is the most common cancer, representing 30% of all recorded cases (Ibrahim, 1986). Schistosomiasis associated bladder cancer differs from bladder cancer in non-endemic areas in two major respects. The peak incidence occurs earlier in life (fourth and fifth decades v. the seventh) and there is a preponderance of squamous cell carcinoma (SCC) rather than TCC (El-Boukainy *et al*, 1972).

In contrast to the situation with TCC, the molecular events underlying tumour development and progression in schistosomiasis associated bladder cancer are not well characterized. Four studies have examined *TP53* mutations in such tumours (Habuchi *et al*, 1993b; Gonzalez-Zulueta *et al*, 1995b; Ramchuuren *et al*, 1995; Warren *et al*, 1995). Mutation frequencies ranged from 33% (Warren *et al*, 1995) to 86% (Habuchi *et al*, 1993b). Since the spectrum of mutations in *TP53* has been shown to reflect the nature of the proposed initiating carcinogen in other tumour types (Greenblatt *et al*, 1994), it is of interest that a significant bias was found in the schistosomiasis tumours towards mutations in exons 5 and 6 and a significantly higher frequency of C→T transitions, most of which were at CpG dinucleotides. It has been suggested that in infected patients this could be induced by nitric oxide produced by inflammatory cells in the bladder wall or by *N*-nitroso compounds generated by bacterial action on nitrates present in the urine. Only a few studies have examined other molecular alterations in these cancers. Ramchuuren *et al* (1995) examined the expression of RB, EGFR and c-ERBB2 proteins by immunohistochemistry and carried out mutation analysis of *HRAS* in 21 SCCs from *S haematobium* infected patients. Three *HRAS* mutations were found and 67 and 28% of tumours showed expression of EGFR and ERBB2 respectively, frequencies similar to those previously reported in TCC specimens (Neal *et al*, 1990; Coombs *et al*, 1991; Levesque *et al*, 1993).

A study by Gonzalez-Zulueta *et al* (1995b) examined chromosome 9 LOH, *CDKN2* homozygous deletion and *TP53* mutation in Egyptian SCCs. Eleven of 19 tumours showed 17p LOH or TP53 immunopositivity, a frequency similar to invasive TCC. Of 9 tumours studied, all had homozygous deletion of *CDKN2* or 9p LOH and all 8 informative cases showed retention of heterozygosity on 9q. This is in stark contrast to the situation in TCC where most cases show LOH of both 9p and 9q.

We have screened 80 bladder cancers obtained from schistosoma infected Egyptian patients for LOH on 12 chromosome arms commonly deleted in TCC (Shaw ME, Elder PA, Abbas A, Knowles MA, unpublished). Our results confirm a striking difference in the frequency of LOH on 9p and 9q with many cases showing 9p LOH (65%) and retention of heterozygosity on 9q. This suggests a major role for *CDKN2/INK4B* in these cancers.

A comparison of the frequency of LOH on selected chromosome arms with that found in TCC is shown in Fig. 4 (Shaw ME, Elder PA, Abbas A, Knowles MA, unpublished). The majority of tumours studied are invasive SCC specimens obtained at cystectomy and the frequencies of 8p LOH, 11q LOH and 17p LOH are reminiscent of those seen in advanced TCC. A comprehensive allelotype of these specimens is now needed to identify novel regions of LOH that may differentiate these tumours from TCC.

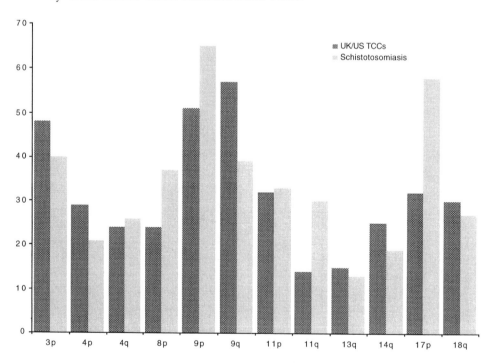

Fig. 4. Comparison of the frequency of LOH on selected chromosome arms in Egyptian schistosomiasis associated bladder cancers (Shaw ME, Elder PA, Abbas A and Knowles MA, unpublished) and TCC (data from Presti *et al*, 1991; Brewster *et al*, 1994; Knowles *et al*, 1994; Chang *et al*, 1995)

A MOLECULAR GENETIC PROGRESSION MODEL FOR TRANSITIONAL CELL CARCINOMA

Does this wealth of genetic information contribute to our understanding of bladder tumour development? As indicated earlier, one of the major problems in determining the molecular progression of bladder tumours is the frequent multifocality of neoplastic change in the bladder. In the past, this led to the concept of "field change" in which it was postulated that exposure of the entire urothelium to carcinogens resulted in the transformation of many cells. The observation of regions of abnormal urothelium ranging from dysplasia to CIS adjacent to overt tumours in the bladder (Schade and Swinney, 1968) has been interpreted as evidence for the proliferation of many clones of altered cells that give rise to multiple tumours either synchronously or metachronously. In an extreme example, each tumour in such a situation might be polyclonal—composed of multiple synchronously evolving clones. At the other extreme, the so called "field change" may represent spread of cells from a single clone so that all tumours in one individual may be monoclonal—all have arisen from a single progenitor cell and have spread through the bladder by a process of intraepithelial migration and/or seeding via the urine. Several molecular studies have attempted to address these possibilities and, as discussed below, present evidence supports both the extreme example of multiple tumours that have evolved from the same precursor cell and situations in which at least two independent clones may have evolved simultaneously. There is no evidence for the existence of polyclonal tumours.

Sidransky *et al* (1992) examined a total of 13 tumours from the cystectomy specimens of four women with multifocal bladder cancer. The pattern of X chromosome inactivation and LOH on chromosome arms 9q, 17p and 18q were studied in all tumours. It was shown that all tumours from the same patient had inactivation of the same X chromosome whereas normal mucosa had random patterns of inactivation, demonstrating that each tumour was monoclonal and that in this small study multifocal tumours in each patient were likely to have arisen from the same precursor cell.

In the same study, it was shown that LOH of 9q in informative patients involved the same allele in all tumours from that patient, suggesting that 9q LOH may have been an early event in the development of these tumours and preceded the spread of the altered clone through the bladder. In contrast, LOH of other chromosome arms did not always affect the same allele, raising the possibility that these events occurred "late" in the genetic evolution of the tumours. A recent study using *TP53* mutations as a marker in multifocal bladder tumours gave similar results to those of Sidransky *et al* for chromosome 9 LOH, with all but one of 17 multifocal tumours from five patients showing the same mutation as the primary tumour (Xu *et al*, 1996). Similarly, a study of a TCC of the renal pelvis and a bladder tumour from the same patient showed identical *TP53* mutations in each case, compatible with seeding of a single clone of altered cells to distant sites in the urinary tract (Lunec *et al*, 1992).

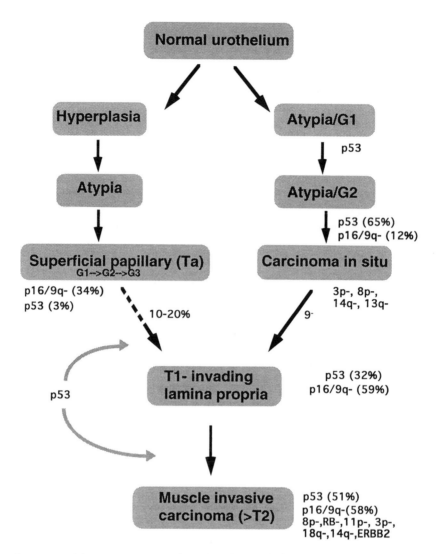

Fig. 5. Model for TCC progression based on histopathological observations and molecular data from references cited in text. Figures in parentheses are observed frequencies reported by Spruck *et al* (1994)

The majority of molecular genetic studies of bladder cancer have examined groups of tumours at one point in their evolution, providing a genetic "snapshot," but no information about the genetic history of the tumour. A histopathological model for the development and progression of bladder cancer predicts two major pathways (Koss *et al*, 1974, 1977) as illustrated in Fig. 5. If we attach to this schema the genetic information that we have, it becomes clear that the molecular findings discussed above are consistent with the previous concept that CIS is a precursor lesion for invasive bladder cancer. Although only a limited number of CIS specimens have been examined in detail, the genetic profile of these is indistinguishable from that of high grade, high stage TCC. This suggests that CIS is genetically an advanced lesion often containing alterations such as *TP53* mutation and LOH of 8p that are demonstrated (*TP53*) or possible (8p-) indicators of poor prognosis.

An interesting study supporting this two pathway model with genetic information (Spruck *et al*, 1994b) showed that in addition to the presence of alterations such as *TP53* mutation at high frequency, CIS/dysplasia differed from papillary tumours by a lower frequency of 9q LOH (12% in CIS compared with 34% in T_a tumours and ≥58% in T_1 and T_2 tumours) indicating CIS is unlikely to be a precursor for papillary TCC. It should be noted, however, that a much higher frequency of 9q LOH was found in the group of CIS specimens examined by Rosin *et al* (1995), which may indicate that there is a significant difference between moderate to severe dysplasia (included in the study of Spruck *et al*) compared with CIS. Spruck *et al* (1994b) analysed several CIS/dysplasia + invasive tumour pairs obtained at the same or different times from the same individual and provided evidence that in some cases progression to an invasive tumour may involve acquisition of alterations to 9q. This result questions the validity of the concept that alterations to chromosome 9 are "early" events in urothelial transformation. If confirmed, it seems that chromosome 9 LOH occurs relatively late in the development of invasive carcinoma via CIS. Possibly, it occurs early in the development of papillary tumours but since we have little or no information about other genetic changes in low grade papillary lesions, nor about the genetics of the low grade hyperplasias/atypias that presumably represent the precursors of these papillary tumours, the only conclusion that can be drawn at present is that chromosome 9 LOH is common by the time a papillary tumour has developed.

A second interesting finding of the study of Spruck *et al* (1994b) was that some of the CIS/dysplasia + invasive tumour pairs studied provided evidence for two independent transformation events. Thus, *TP53* mutations present in the CIS were not always present in the invasive tumour from the same patient or a different *TP53* mutation was found. Similar findings have now been reported by Chaturvedi *et al* (1997) who also showed that *TP53* mutation is present not only in CIS but also in low grade dysplasia present in cystectomy specimens. As yet, the timing of *TP53* mutation in the few superficial papillary tumours that progress to muscle invasion has not been investigated directly, but it can be inferred from the observed frequencies in T_a, T_1 and T_2 tumours (Spruck *et al*, 1994b) that this may happen at the stage of invasion of the lamina propria or muscle.

These results indicate that within the same bladder a single clone may evolve by the acquisition of different genetic changes to give rise to multiple tumours that may share certain genetic alterations but may also differ in several ways. They also provide evidence that more than one initiating event may occur in the bladder. This could now be tested in a more extensive series of female patients using X chromosome inactivation to identify different clones. It is likely that clones that have acquired particularly advantageous characteristics such as

TP53 mutations may predominate, so that the apparently simple results obtained from cystectomy specimens, which by definition will contain an aggressively neoplastic clone, may not be representative of the situation in the bladder at an earlier stage of the disease, with a single or several papillary low grade non-invasive tumours. This of course is the situation that is inherently more interesting, since it offers the opportunity for choices in clinical intervention. Clearly, larger studies involving multiple genetic markers will be needed to understand the situation more fully.

SUMMARY AND FUTURE DIRECTIONS

Already several genetic alterations promise to have clinical application. These include the use of *TP53* and *RB* inactivation to predict rapid clinical progression and possibly in the case of *TP53*, response to chemotherapy. These and a range of alterations identified in muscle invasive tumours require careful assessment as possible markers of progression in superficial bladder cancer and this will initially require large retrospective studies on patients for whom complete clinical follow up information is available. Steps have already been taken to use genetic markers to screen urine from patients at presentation and the success rate in identifying the presence of a tumour is encouragingly high (Mao *et al*, 1996). Similarly, once a tumour has been resected, specific genetic changes identified in the tumour can be applied to the non-invasive monitoring of the disease in urine samples. *TP53* mutations have been used in this way and extremely promising results obtained (Xu *et al*, 1996). For example, specific mutations have been detected in patients after resection in whom no obvious tumour recurrence was apparent, indicating the continued presence of altered cells in the "normal" urothelium and suggesting the need for increased vigilance in such patients.

Several genetic alterations have shown no obvious association with tumour grade or stage. As we identify more of the genes involved and our understanding of the cellular processes in which they participate increases, it is likely that groups of genes involved in the same pathway may together be found to have more predictive power than any single gene. In the future, we will also have the ability to study these markers on very precisely dissected specimens comprising a few cells, for example using the technique of laser capture microdissection (Emmert-Buck *et al*, 1996).

Our understanding of the genetics of bladder cancer, particularly TCC, has advanced greatly during the past decade. We now know many of the components of the genotype of invasive bladder cancer and the challenge now is to build models using these which will give mechanistic insight and have clinical power. Already a great deal of information about the phenotypic effects of certain genetic alterations has come from the in vitro model of human urothelial cell transformation developed by Reznikoff and co-workers (1996). Interestingly, several of the alterations that accompany spontaneous progression of immortal human urothelial cells in vitro parallel what is seen in tumour specimens. Development of this model using specific gene knockouts and the introduction of oncogenes implicated in TCC in vivo will be a valuable step in applying knowledge we have acquired from tumour material.

In vivo models of urothelial tumour development are also needed. These might involve specific transgenic or knockout animals, but a more powerful approach is likely to involve the reconstruction of urothelium in vivo from genetically manipulated cells as has been achieved so successfully for mouse mammary tissue and prostate (Edwards, 1993; Thompson *et al*, 1993). A preliminary study involving heterotransplantation under the kidney capsule of mouse bladder cells, into which viral MYC and SRC oncogenes had been introduced alone or in combination, yielded very promising results, with the development of dysplasia in the reconstituted tissue from the manipulated cells (Wagner *et al*, 1990). In such systems there is the clear advantage that genetically altered cells are able to interact with their normal counterparts, or other cells, a situation that is likely to be vital if we are to understand the dynamics of preneoplasia and tumour progression in the bladder.

Another key area for future work is to identify genetic alterations in superficial papillary tumours. These represent the largest group of bladder tumours, about which we know virtually nothing save for the involvement of chromosome 9 alterations. This is likely to require novel approaches such as the use of comparative genomic hybridization (Kallioniemi *et al*, 1992) to search for gene amplifications, the application of representational difference analysis (Lisitsyn *et al*, 1993) to search for small regions of homozygous deletion and techniques such as differential display (Liang and Pardee, 1992) or DNA chip technologies (Schena *et al*, 1995; Velculescu *et al*, 1995) to explore alterations in gene expression. Molecular genetic studies of cancer to date have identfed three classes of genes involved, the oncogenes, the tumour suppressor genes and genes that maintain genome integrity. It is likely that in the next few years our horizons will broaden to take into account the role of genes that influence, for example, the interactions of a cell with surrounding cells and the intercellular matrix, which influence angiogenesis or recognition by the immune system.

Acknowledgements

Work in the author's laboratory has been funded by Marie Curie Cancer Care and by grants from the Medical Research Council and Association for International Cancer Research.

References

Bell D, Taylor JA, Paulson DF, Robertson CN, Mohler JL and Lucier GW (1993) Genetic risk and carcinogen exposure: a common inherited defect of the carcinogen-metabolism gene glutathione S-transferase M1 (GSTM1) that increases susceptibility to bladder cancer. *Journal of the National Cancer Institute* **85** 1159–1164

Bell SM, Zuo J, Myers RM and Knowles MA (1996) Fluorescence in situ hybridization deletion mapping at 4p16.3 in bladder cancer cell lines refines the localization of the critical interval to 30kb. *Genes, Chromosomes and Cancer* **17** 108–117

Bell SM, Shaw M, Jou Y-S, Myers RM and Knowles MA (1997) Identification and characterization of the human homologue of SH3BP2, an SH3 binding domain protein within a common region of deletion at 4p16.3 involved in bladder cancer. *Genomics* (in press)

Bergerheim USR, Kunimi K, Collins VP and Ekman P (1991) Deletion mapping on chromosomes 8, 10 and 16 in human prostatic carcinoma. *Genes, Chromosomes and Cancer* **3** 215–220

Brewster SF, Gingell JC, Browne S and Brown KW (1994) Loss of heterozygosity on chromosome 18q is associated with muscle-invasive transitional cell carcinoma of the bladder. *British Journal of Cancer* **70** 697–700

Bringuier PP, Tamimi J and Schuuring E (1994) Amplification of the chromosome 11q13 region in bladder tumours. *Urological Research* **21** 451

Bringuier PP, Tamimi Y, Schuuring E and Schalken J (1996) Expression of cyclin D1 and EMS1 in bladder tumours: relationship with chromosome 11q13 amplification. *Oncogene* **12** 1747–1753

Brockmoller J, Kerb R, Drakoulis N, Staffeldt B and Roots I (1995) Glutathione S-transferase M1 and its variants A and B as host factors of bladder cancer susceptibility: a case-control study. *Cancer Research* **54** 4103–4111

Cairns P, Proctor AJ and Knowles MA (1991) Loss of heterozygosity at the *RB* locus is frequent and correlates with muscle invasion in bladder carcinoma. *Oncogene* **6** 2305–2309

Cairns P, Shaw ME and Knowles MA (1993a) Initiation of bladder cancer may involve deletion of a tumour-suppressor gene on chromosome 9. *Oncogene* **8** 1083–1085

Cairns P, Shaw ME and Knowles MA (1993b) Preliminary mapping of the deleted region of chromosome 9 in bladder cancer. *Cancer Research* **53** 1230–1232

Cairns P, Tokino K, Eby Y and Sidransky D (1994) Homozygous deletions of 9p21 in primary human bladder tumors detected by comparative multiplex polymerase chain reaction. *Cancer Research* **54** 1422–1424

Cairns P, Polascik TJ, Eby Y *et al* (1995) Frequency of homozygous deletion at *p16/CDKN2* in primary human tumours. *Nature Genetics* **11** 210–212

Carbonara C, Longa L, Grosso E *et al* (1994) 9q34 loss of heterozygosity in a tuberous sclerosis astrocytoma suggests a growth suppressor-like activity also for the TSC1 gene. *Human Molecular Genetics* **3** 1829–1832

Cartwright RA, Glashan RW, Rogers HJ *et al* (1982) The role of N-acetyltransferase in bladder carcinogenesis: a pharmacogenetic epidemiological approach to bladder cancer. *Lancet* **ii** 842–846

Chang WY-H, Cairns P, Schoenberg MP, Polascik TJ and Sidransky D (1995) Novel suppressor loci on chromosome 14q in primary bladder cancer. *Cancer Research* **55** 3246–3249

Chaturvedi V, Li L, Hodges S *et al* (1997) Superimposed histologic and genetic mapping of chromosome 17 alterations in human urinary bladder neoplasia. *Oncogene* **14** 2059–2070

Cook PJ, Doll R and Fellingham S (1969) A mathematical model for the age distribution of cancer in man. *International Journal of Cancer* **4** 93–112

Coombs LM, Piggott DA, Sweeney E *et al* (1991) Amplification and overexpression of c-*erb*B-2 in transitional cell carcinoma of the urinary bladder. *British Journal of Cancer* **63** 601–608

Cordon-Cardo C, Wartinger D, Petrylak D *et al* (1992) Altered expression of the retinoblastoma gene product: prognostic indicator in bladder cancer. *Journal of the National Cancer Institute* **84** 1251–1256

Cordon-Cardo C, Dalbagni G, Saez GT *et al* (1994) TP53 mutations in human bladder cancer: genotypic versus phenotypic patterns. *International Journal of Cancer* **56** 347–353

Cordon-Cardo C, Zhang Z-F, Dalbagni G *et al* (1997) Cooperative effects of p53 and pRB alterations in primary superficial bladder tumors. *Cancer Research* **57** 1217–1221

Cote RJ, Esrig D, Groshen S, Jones PA and Skinner DG (1997) p53 and treatment of bladder cancer. *Nature* **385** 123–125

Dalbagni G, Presti J, Reuter V, Fair WR and Cordon-Cardo C (1993) Genetic alterations in bladder cancer. *Lancet* **342** 469–471

Devlin J, Keen AJ and Knowles MA (1994) Homozygous deletion mapping at 9p21 in bladder carcinoma defines a critical region within 2cM of *IFNA*. *Oncogene* **9** 2757–2760

Edwards PAW (1993) Tissue reconstitution models of breast cancer. In Lemoine NR and Wright NA (eds). *Cancer Surveys* vol. 16 *Breast Cancer* pp 79–96 Cold Spring Harbor Laboratory Press, Cold Spring Harbor, New York

El-Boukainy MN, Ghoneim MA and Mansour MA (1972) Carcinoma of bilharzial bladder in Egypt: clinical and pathological features. *British Journal of Urology* **44** 561–570

Elder PA, Bell SM and Knowles MA (1994) Deletion of two regions on chromosome 4 in bladder carcinoma: definition of a critical 750kb region at 4p16.3. *Oncogene* **9** 3433–3436

Emi M, Fujiwara Y, Ohata H *et al* (1993) Allelic loss at chromosome band 8p21.3-p22 is associated with progression of hepatocellular carcinoma. *Genes, Chromosomes and Cancer* **7** 152–157

Emmert-Buck MR, Bonner RF, Smith PD *et al* (1996) Laser capture microdissection. *Science* **274** 998–1001

Esrig D, Elmajian D, Groshen S *et al* (1994) Accumulation of nuclear p53 and tumor progression in bladder cancer. *New England Journal of Medicine* **331** 1259–1264

Eydmann ME and Knowles MA (1997) Mutation analysis of 8p genes *POLB* and *PPP2CB* in bladder cancer. *Cancer Genetics and Cytogenetics* **93** 167–171

Fearon ER, Feinberg AP, Hamilton SH and Vogelstein B (1985) Loss of genes on the short arm of chromosome 11 in bladder cancer. *Nature* **318** 377–380

Fitzgerald JM, Ramchurren N, Rieger K *et al* (1995) Identification of H-*ras* mutations in urine sediments complements cytology in the detection of bladder tumors. *Journal of the National Cancer Institute* **87** 129–133

Fujimoto K, Yamada Y, Okajima E *et al* (1992) Frequent association of p53 gene mutation in invasive bladder cancer. *Cancer Research* **52** 1393–1398

Fujita J, Srivastava SK, Kraus MH, Rhim JS, Tronick SR and Aaronson SA (1985) Frequency of molecular alterations affecting *ras* protooncogenes in human urinary tract tumors. *Proceedings of the National Academy of Sciences of the USA* **82** 3849–3853

Fujiwara Y, Emi M, Ohata H *et al* (1993) Evidence for the presence of two tumor suppressor genes on chromosome 8p for colorectal carcinoma. *Cancer Research* **53** 1172–1174

Gonzalez-Zulueta M, Ruppert JM, Tokino K *et al* (1993) Microsatellite instability in bladder cancer. *Cancer Research* **53** 5620–5623

Gonzalez-Zulueta M, Bender CM, Yang AS *et al* (1995a) Methylation of the 5′ CpG island of the *p16/CDKN2* tumor suppressor gene in normal and transformed human tissues correlates with gene silencing. *Cancer Research* **55** 4531–4535

Gonzalez-Zulueta M, Shibata A, Ohneseit PF *et al* (1995b) High frequency of chromosome 9p allelic loss and *CDKN2* tumor suppressor gene alterations in squamous cell carcinoma of the bladder. *Journal of the National Cancer Institute* **87** 1383–1393

Green AJ, Johnson PH and Yates JRW (1994) The tuberous sclerosis gene on chromosome 9q34 acts as a growth suppressor. *Human Molecular Genetics* **3** 1833–1834

Greenblatt MS, Bennett WP, Hollstein M and Harris CC (1994) Mutations in the p53 tumor suppressor gene: clues to cancer etiology and molecular pathogenesis. *Cancer Research* **54** 4855–4878

Gruis NA, Weaver-Feldhaus J, Liu Q *et al* (1995) Genetic evidence in melanoma and bladder cancers that p16 and p53 function in separate pathways of tumor suppression. *American Journal of Pathology* **146** 1199–1206

Habuchi T, Ogawa O, Kakehi Y *et al* (1993a) Accumulated allelic losses in the development of invasive urothelial cancer. *International Journal of Cancer* **53** 579–584

Habuchi T, Takahashi R, Yamada H *et al* (1993b) Influence of cigarette smoking and schistoso-miasis on p53 gene mutation in urothelial cancer. *Cancer Research* **53** 3795–3799

Habuchi T, Kinoshita H, Yamada H *et al* (1994) Oncogene amplification in urothelial cancers with p53 gene mutation or MDM2 amplification. *Journal of the National Cancer Institute* **86** 1331–1335

Habuchi T, Devlin J, Elder PA and Knowles MA (1995) Detailed deletion mapping of chromo-some 9q in bladder cancer: evidence for two tumour suppressor loci. *Oncogene* **11** 1671–1674

Habuchi T, Yoshida O and Knowles MA (1997) A novel candidate tumour suppressor locus at 9q32-33 in bladder cancer: localisation of the candidate region within a single 840kb YAC. *Human Molecular Genetics* **6** 913–919

Hussussian CJ, Struewing JP, Goldstein AM *et al* (1994) Germline mutations in familial melanoma. *Nature Genetics* **8** 15–21

IARC (1994) Schistosomes, liver flukes and *Helicobacter pylori*. IARC *Monographs on the Evaluation of Carcinogenic Risks to Humans* **61**

Ibrahim SA (1986) Site distribution of cancer in Egypt: twelve years' experience (1970–1981), In: Ismail A (ed.) *Cancer Prevention in Developing Countries*, pp. 45–50, Pergamon, Oxford

Ishikawa J, Xu H-J, Hu S-X *et al* (1991) Inactivation of the retinoblastoma gene in human blad-der and renal cell carcinomas. *Cancer Research* **51** 5736–5743

Kallioniemi A, Kallioniemi O-P, Sudar D *et al* (1992) Comparative genomic hybridization for mol-ecular genetic analysis of solid tumors. *Science* **258** 818–821

Kallioniemi A, Kallioniemi O-P, Citro G *et al* (1995) Identification of gains and losses of DNA sequences in primary bladder cancer by comparative genomic hybridization. *Genes, Chromosomes and Cancer* **12** 213–219

Kamb A, Gruis NA, Weaver-Feldhaus J *et al* (1994) A cell cycle regulator potentially involved in genesis of many tumor types. *Science* **264** 436–440

Kantor AF, Hartge P, Hoover RN and Fraumeni JF Jr (1985) Familial and environmental inter-actions in bladder cancer risk. *International Journal of Cancer* **35** 703–706

Keen AJ and Knowles MA (1994) Definition of two regions of deletion on chromosome 9 in car-cinoma of the bladder. *Oncogene* **9** 2083–2088

Klingelhutz A, Wu S-Q, Bookland E and Reznikoff C (1991) Allelic 3p deletions in high grade carcinomas after transformation in vitro of human uroepithelial cells. *Genes, Chromosomes and Cancer* **3** 346–357

Knowles MA, Shaw ME and Proctor AJ (1993) Deletion mapping of chromosome 8 in cancers of the urinary bladder using restriction fragment length polymorphisms and microsatellite poly-morphisms. *Oncogene* **8** 1357–1364

Knowles MA, Elder PA, Williamson M, Cairns JP, Shaw ME and Law M (1994) Allelotype of human bladder cancer. *Cancer Research* **54** 531–538

Koss LG (1975) *Atlas of Tumor Pathology: Tumors of the Urinary Bladder (Fascicle 11)*, 2nd ed, Washington DC: Armed Forces Institute of Pathology

Koss LG (1979) Mapping of the urinary bladder: its impact on the concepts of bladder cancer. *Human Pathology* **10** 533–548

Koss LG, Tiamson EM and Robbins MA (1974) Mapping cancerous and precancerous bladder changes. A study of the urothelium in ten surgically removed bladders. *Journal of the American Medical Association* **227** 281–286

Koss LG, Nakanishi I and Freed SZ (1977) Nonpapillary carcinoma *in situ* and atypical hyper-plasia in cancerous bladders: further studies of surgically removed bladders by mapping. *Urology* **9** 442–455

Lamm DL (1992) Carcinoma *in situ*. *Urology Clinics of North America* **19** 499–508

Levesque P, Ramchuuren N, Saini K, Joyce A, Libertino J and Summerhayes IC (1993) Screening of human bladder tumors and urine sediments for the presence of H-*ras* mutations. *International Journal of Cancer* **55** 785–790

Lianes P, Orlow I, Zhang Z-F *et al* (1994) Altered patterns of MDM2 and TP53 expression in human bladder cancer. *Journal of the National Cancer Institute* **86** 1325–1330

Liang P and Pardee AB (1992) Differential display of eukaryotic messenger RNA by means of the polymerase chain reaction. *Science* **257** 967–971

Lipponen PK (1993) Over-expression of p53 nuclear oncoprotein in transitional-cell bladder cancer and its prognostic value. *International Journal of Cancer* **53** 365–370

Lisitsyn N, Lisitsyn N and Wigler M (1993) Cloning the differences between complex genomes. *Science* **259** 946–951

Logothetis CJ, Xu H-J, Ro JY *et al* (1992) Altered expression of retinoblastoma protein and known prognostic variables in locally advanced bladder cancer. *Journal of the National Cancer Institute* **84** 1256–1261

Lowe SW, Ruley HE, Jacks T and Housman DE (1993) p53-dependent apoptosis modulates the cytotoxicity of anticancer agents. *Cell* **74** 957–967

Lunec J, Challen C, Wright C, Mellon K and Neal DE (1992) c-erbB-2 amplification and identical p53 mutations in concomitant transitional carcinomas of renal pelvis and urinary bladder. *Lancet* **339** 439–440

Lynch HT, Walzak MP, Fried R, Domina AH and Lynch JF (1979) Familial factors in bladder carcinoma. *Journal of Urology* **122** 458–461

Lynch HT, Kimberling WJ, Lynch JF and Brennan K (1987) Familial bladder cancer in an oncology clinic. *Cancer Genetics and Cytogenetics* **27** 161–165

McCullough DL, Lamm DL, McLaughlin AP III and Gittes RF (1975) Familial transitional cell carcinoma of the bladder. *Journal of Urology* **113** 629–639

Malone PR, Visvinathan KV, Ponder BAJ, Shearer RJ and Summerhayes IC (1985) Oncogenes and bladder cancer. *British Journal of Urology* **57** 664–667

Mao L, Schoenberg MP, Scicchitano M *et al* (1996) Molecular detection of primary bladder cancer by microsatellite analysis. *Science* **271** 659–662

Mellon JK, Lunec J, Wright C, Horne CH, Kelly P and Neal DE (1996) C-ERBB-2 in bladder cancer: molecular biology, correlation with epidermal growth factor receptors and prognostic value. *Journal of Urology* **155** 321–326

Miyamoto H, Shuin T, Torigoe S, Iwasaki Y and Kubota Y (1995) Retinoblastoma gene mutations in primary human bladder cancer. *British Journal of Cancer* **71** 831–835

Miyao N, Tsai YC, Lerner SP *et al* (1993) Role of chromosome 9 in human bladder cancer. *Cancer Research* **53** 4066–4070

Neal DE, Sharples L, Smith K, Fenelly J, Hall RR and Harris AL (1990) The epidermal growth factor receptor and the prognosis of bladder cancer. *Cancer* **65** 1619–1625

Nobori T, Miura K, Wu DJ, Lois A, Takabayashi K and Carson DA (1994) Deletions of the cyclin-dependent kinase-4 inhibitor gene in multiple human cancers. *Nature* **368** 753–756

Olumi AF, Tsai YC, Nichols PW *et al* (1990) Allelic loss of chromosome 17p distinguishes high grade from low grade transitional cell carcinomas of the bladder. *Cancer Research* **50** 7081–7083

Ooi A, Herz F, Ii S *et al* (1994) Ha-*ras* codon 12 mutation in papillary tumors of the urinary bladder: a retrospective study. *International Journal of Oncology* **4** 85–90

Orlow I, Lacombe L, Hannon GJ *et al* (1995) Deletion of the p16 and p15 genes in human bladder tumors. *Journal of the National Cancer Institute* **87** 1524–1529

Perucho M (1997) Cancer of the microsatellite mutator phenotype. *Biological Chemistry* **11** 675–684

Polascik TJ, Cairns P, Chang WYH, Schoenberg MP and Sidransky D (1995) Distinct regions of allelic loss on chromosome 4 in human primary bladder carcinoma. *Cancer Research* **55** 5396–5399

Pratt CI, Kao C, Wu S-Q, Gilchrist KW, Oyasu R and Reznikoff CA (1992) Neoplastic progression by EJ/*ras* at different steps of transformation *in vitro* of human uroepithelial cells. *Cancer Research* **52** 688–695

Presti JC Jr, Reuter VE, Galan T, Fair WR and Cordon-Cardo C (1991) Molecular genetic alterations in superficial and locally advanced human bladder cancer. *Cancer Research* **51** 5405–5409

Proctor AJ, Coombs LM, Cairns JP and Knowles MA (1991) Amplification at chromosome 11q13 in transitional cell tumours of the bladder. *Oncogene* **6** 789–795

Ramchuuren N, Cooper K and Summerhayes IC (1995) Molecular events underlying schistosomiasis-related bladder cancer. *International Journal of Cancer* **62** 237–244

Reznikoff CA, Belair CD, Yeager TR *et al* (1996) A molecular genetic model of human bladder cancer pathogenesis. *Seminars in Oncology* **5** 571–584

Risch A, Wallace DMA, Bathers S and Sim E (1995) Slow N-acetylation genotype is a susceptibility factor in occupational and smoking related bladder cancer. *Human Molecular Genetics* **4** 231–236

Rosin MP, Cairns P, Epstein JI, Schoenberg MP and Sidransky D (1995) Partial allelotype of carcinoma *in situ* of the human bladder. *Cancer Research* **55** 5213–5216

Ruppert JM, Tokino K and Sidransky D (1993) Evidence for two bladder cancer suppressor loci on human chromosome 9. *Cancer Research* **53** 5093–5095

Sandberg AA and Berger CS (1994) Review of chromosome studies in urological tumors. II. Cytogenetics and molecular genetics of bladder cancer. *Journal of Urology* **151** 545–560

Sarkis AS, Dalbagni G, Cordon-Cardo C *et al* (1993a) Nuclear overexpression of p53 protein in transitional cell bladder carcinoma: a marker for disease progression. *Journal of the National Cancer Institute* **85** 53–59

Sarkis AS, Zhang Z-F, Cordon-Cardo C *et al* (1993b) p53 nuclear overexpression and disease progression in Ta bladder carcinoma. *International Journal of Oncology* **3** 355–360

Sarkis AS, Dalbagni G, Cordon-Cardo C *et al* (1994) Association of p53 nuclear overexpression and tumor progression in carcinoma in situ of the bladder. *Journal of Urology* **152** 388–392

Sato K, Moriyama M, Mori S *et al* (1992) An immunohistologic evaluation of c-erbB-2 gene product in patients with urinary bladder carcinoma. *Cancer* **70** 2493–2498

Sauter G, Moch H, Moore D *et al* (1993) Heterogeneity of erbB-2 gene amplification in bladder cancer. *Cancer Research* **53** 2199–2203

Schade ROK and Swinney J (1968) Pre-cancerous changes in bladder epithelium. *Lancet* **ii** 943–946

Schena M, Shalon D, Davis R and Brown P (1995) Quantitative monitoring of gene expression patterns with a complementary DNA microarray. *Science* **270** 467–470

Shapiro GI, Edwards CD, Kobzik L *et al* (1995) Reciprocal Rb inactivation and p16INK4 expression in primary lung cancers and cell lines. *Cancer Research* **55** 505–509

Shaw ME and Knowles MA (1995) Deletion mapping of chromosome 11 in carcinoma of the bladder. *Genes, Chromosomes and Cancer* **13** 1–8

Sidransky D, von Eschenbach A, Tsai YC *et al* (1991) Identification of p53 gene mutations in bladder cancers and urine samples. *Science* **252** 706–709

Sidransky D, Frost P, von Eschenbach A, Oyasu R, Preisinger AC and Vogelstein B (1992) Clonal origin of bladder cancer. *New England Journal of Medicine* **326** 737–740

Sigalas I, Calvert AH, Anderson JJ, Neal DE and Lunec J (1996) Alternatively spliced *mdm2* transcripts with loss of p53 binding domain sequences: transforming ability and frequent detection in human cancer. *Nature Medicine* **2** 912–917

Simoneau AR, Spruck CH III, Gonzalez-Zulueta M *et al* (1996) Evidence for two tumor suppressor loci associated with proximal chromosome 9p to q and distal chromosome 9q in bladder cancer and the initial screening for *GAS1* and *PTC* mutations. *Cancer Research* **56** 5039–5043

Soini Y, Turpeenniemi-Hujanen T, Kamel D *et al* (1993) p53 immunohistochemistry in transitional cell carcinoma and dysplasia of the urinary bladder correlates with disease progression. *British Journal of Cancer* **68** 1029–1035

Spruck CH III, Rideout WM III, Olumi AF *et al* (1993) Distinct pattern of p53 mutations in bladder cancer: relationship to tobacco usage. *Cancer Research* **53** 1162–1166

Spruck CH III, Gonzalez-Zulueta M, Shibata A *et al* (1994a) p16 gene in uncultured tumours. *Nature* **370** 183–184

Spruck CH III, Ohneseit PF, Gonzalez-Zulueta M *et al* (1994b) Two molecular pathways to transitional cell carcinoma of the bladder. *Cancer Research* **54** 784–788

Takle LA and Knowles MA (1996) Deletion mapping implicates two tumour suppressor genes on chromosome 8p in the development of bladder cancer. *Oncogene* **12** 1083–1087

Theodorescu D, Cornil I, Sheehan C, Man MS and Kerbel RS (1991) Ha-*ras* induction of the invasive phenotype results in up-regulation of epidermal growth factor receptors and altered responsiveness to epidermal growth factor in human papillary transitional cell carcinoma cells. *Cancer Research* **51** 4486–4491

Thompson TC, Truong LD, Timme TL *et al* (1993) Transgenic models for the study of prostate cancer. *Cancer* **71** 1165–1171

Tsai YC, Nichols PW, Hiti AL *et al* (1990) Allelic losses of chromosomes 9, 11 and 17 in human bladder cancer. *Cancer Research* **50** 44–47

Underwood M, Bartlett J, Reeves J, Gardiner S, Scott R and Cooke T (1995) C-*erbB*-2 gene amplification: a molecular marker in recurrent bladder tumors? *Cancer Research* **55** 2422–2430

van Slegtenhorst M, de Hoogt T, Hermans C *et al.* (1997) Identification of the tuberous sclerosis gene TSC1 on chromosome 9q34. *Science* **277** 805–808

Velculescu VE, Zhang L, Vogelstein B and Kinzler KW (1995) Serial analysis of gene expression. *Science* **270** 484–487

Voorter CEM, Ummelin MIJ, Ramaekers FSC and Hopman AHN (1996) Loss of chromosome 11 and 11P/Q imbalances in bladder cancer detected by fluorescence *in situ* hybridisation. *International Journal of Cancer* **65** 301–307

Wagner HE, Steele G Jr and Summerhayes IC (1990) Preneoplastic lesions induced by myc and src oncogenes in reconstituted mouse bladder. *Surgery* **108** 146–152

Wagner U, Sauter G, Moch H *et al* (1995) Patterns of p53, erbB-2 and EGF-r expression in premalignant lesions of the urinary bladder. *Human Pathology* **26** 970–978

Waldman T, Lengauer C, Kinzler KW and Vogelstein B (1996) Uncoupling of S phase and mitosis by anticancer agents in cells lacking p21. *Science* **381** 713–716

Warren W, Biggs PJ, El-Baz M, Ghoneim MA, Stratton MR and Venitt S (1995) Mutations in the p53 gene in schistosomal bladder cancer: a study of 92 tumors from Egyptian patients and a comparison between spectra from schistosomal and non-schistosomal urothelial tumors. *Carcinogenesis* **16** 1181–1189

WHO (1985) *The Control of Schistosomiasis. Report of a WHO Expert Committee.* Geneva: World Health Organization

Williams B, Remington L, Albert D, Mukai S, Bronson R and Jacks T (1994) Cooperative tumorigenic effects of germline mutations in Rb and p53. *Nature Genetics* **7** 480–484

Williamson MP, Elder PA and Knowles MA (1994) The spectrum of *TP53* mutations in bladder carcinoma. *Genes, Chromosomes and Cancer* **9** 108–118

Williamson MP, Elder PA, Shaw ME, Devlin J and Knowles MA (1995) p16 (*CDKN2*) is a major deletion target at 9p21 in bladder cancer. *Human Molecular Genetics* **4** 1569–1577

Wu Q, Possati L, Montesi M *et al* (1996) Growth arrest and suppression of tumorigenicity of bladder carcinoma cell lines induced by the *p16/CDKN2* (*p16INK4A, MTS1*) gene and other loci on chromosome 9. *International Journal of Cancer* **65** 840–846

Xu H-J, Cairns P, Hu S-X, Knowles MA and Benedict WF (1993) Loss of RB protein expression in primary bladder cancer correlates with loss of heterozygosity at the RB locus and tumor progression. *International Journal of Cancer* **53** 781–784

Xu X, Stower MJ, Reid IN, Garner RC and Burns PA (1996) Molecular screening of multifocal transitional cell carcinoma of the bladder using *p53* mutations as biomarkers. *Clinical Cancer Research* **2** 1795–1800

Yeager T, Stadler W, Belair C, Puthenveettil J, Olopade O and Reznikoff C (1995) Increased p16 levels correlate with pRB alterations in human urothelial cells. *Cancer Research* **55** 493–497

Zhau HE, Zhang X, von Eschenbach AC, Scorsone K and Hung M-C (1990) Amplification and expression of c-erbB-2 in transitional cell carcinoma of the urinary bladder. *Molecular Carcinogenesis* **3** 254–257

The author is responsible for the accuracy of the references.

Molecular Biological Changes in Bladder Cancer

KHAVER N QURESHI[1] • JOHN LUNEC[2] • DAVID E NEAL[1]

[1]*Department of Surgery; and* [2]*Cancer Research Unit, University of Newcastle, Newcastle upon Tyne NE2 4HH*

Introduction
Conventional grading and staging
Oncogenes and bladder cancer
    RAS
    MYC
    JUN
Epidermal growth factor receptor family
    Epidermal growth factor receptor
    ERBB2
Loss of heterozygosity studies
Cell cycle and retinoblastoma
***TP53* tumour suppressor gene and bladder cancer**
    CDKN1A and *TP53*
    MDM2 and *TP53*
    BCL2, *BAX* and *TP53* mediated apoptosis
Metalloproteinases
Angiogenesis
Cell adhesion molecules
Summary

INTRODUCTION

A major issue in the management of bladder cancer is the prediction of prognosis and survival. Most patients with superficial bladder cancer (pT_a and pT_1) have a good prognosis, although 50–70% develop recurrences and 10–25% may progress to muscle invasive or metastatic disease. Patients with muscle invasive disease have only a 50% two year survival despite treatment. The difficulty of explaining and predicting future tumour behaviour has spurred the identification of genetic alterations. The identification of such changes has potential benefits not only for the prediction of disease progression and treatment response but also for providing insight into mechanisms relevant to human bladder cancer and the identification of new treatment approaches.

CONVENTIONAL GRADING AND STAGING

Transitional cell carcinoma (TCC) is the most common histological type of bladder cancer. The pathological appearance ranges from a solitary superficial papillary lesion to an extensive tumour with invasion of contiguous viscera and distant metastasis. The evolution of histological grading and staging systems for bladder cancer has stemmed from the observations of the clinical course of different tumours in association with their depth of penetration through the bladder wall.

Staging of bladder cancer is based on the TNM system. Approximately 75% of bladder tumours present as superficial (non-invasive) TCC (T_{is}, T_a and T_1), and the remainder are muscle invasive TCCs (T_2, T_{3a}, T_{3b}, T_{4a} and T_{4b}). Tumours that are restricted to the mucosa with no lamina propria invasion are classified as T_a and flat carcinoma-in-situ (CIS). T_1 tumours have penetrated the lamina propria but not the muscle. Muscle invasive tumours account for 20% of newly diagnosed TCCs and usually present de novo rather than developing from previous superficial lesions. Superficial and deep muscle invasion are staged as T_2 and T_{3a}, respectively. Invasion of perivesical fat is denoted as T_{3b}, and invasion of prostate or vagina is T_{4a}. T_{4b} refers to a tumour that is fixed to the pelvis or abdominal wall (Fig. 1). Lymph node involvement is classified as N_1 to N_4 and distant metastasis as M_0 or M_1 (Mostofi *et al*, 1973).

Pathological grading of TCCs closely correlates with the stage of the disease (Kern, 1984). Grading of tumours is based on histological characteristics, including nuclear abnormalities, extent of differentiation, increased mitotic activity, deranged microscopical architecture and anaplasia. Using this information tumours can be graded as low, medium or high grade (G_1, G_2 or G_3).

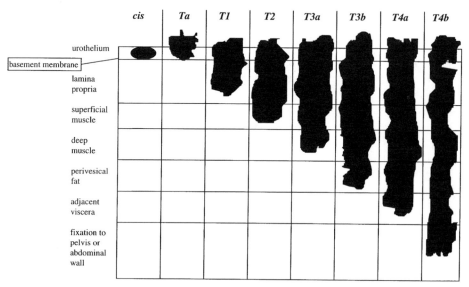

Fig. 1. Staging of bladder tumours. *cis* = carcinoma in situ

The best predictor of survival is clinical stage, followed by histological grade (Narayana *et al*, 1983). However, other features are informative, such as the presence of concomitant carcinoma-in-situ, tumour type (papillary/solid), tumour size and number, vascular invasion, age of the patient and location of the tumour (Liebert and Seigne, 1996). Of the established prognostic indicators, none is specific or sensitive enough to identify precisely those patients in whom early radical therapy would be beneficial or to distinguish patients who would benefit from intervention (surgery, chemotherapy or radiotherapy). To address this problem investigators have turned to molecular biology in the hope that molecular markers may provide diagnostic and prognostic information to aid the clinician in treating patients with bladder cancer. These molecular pathology studies also test the relevance of mechanisms established in in vitro model systems and identify novel therapeutic targets.

ONCOGENES AND BLADDER CANCER

RAS

The human *RAS* gene family consists of three closely related and highly conserved genes: *HRAS*, *KRAS* and *NRAS*. The related gene products are membrane associated 21 kDa GTP binding proteins, whose normal functions are in growth signal transduction from cell surface growth factor receptors. The activation of the proto-oncogene is by point mutation, and *HRAS* mutations have been demonstrated in 18% of primary bladder tumours, detected by direct polymerase chain reaction (PCR) sequencing. No correlation was shown with tumour grade or stage, which suggests that this is an early event in the development of bladder cancer (Burchill *et al*, 1994). In contrast, *HRAS* mutations were present in only 6% of bladder tumours when assessed by single strand conformation polymorphism (SSCP) (Knowles and Williamson, 1995). With SSCP analysis, mutations in exon 1 of the *HRAS* gene were detected in urine sediments from 44% of patients with primary bladder tumours (Fitzgerald *et al*, 1995). This method was significantly more sensitive in detecting low grade (G_{1-2}) lesions than conventional cytological methods, although the latter was more effective in identifying CIS. The combined use of these two techniques resulted in a 1.8-fold increase in tumour detection rate compared with the use of urine cytology alone.

MYC

Members of the *MYC* gene family are important regulators of cell proliferation. They encode nuclear phosphoproteins involved in transcriptional regulation. The *MYC* oncogene maps to chromosome 8q. High expression of *MYC* detected immunohistochemically has been associated with poorly differentiated tumours (Kotake *et al*, 1990), and cytoplasmic immunoreactivity was found to correlate with histological grade, papillary configuration, S phase fraction, mitotic index and overexpression of epidermal growth factor receptor (EGFR), although it had no prognostic value in survival analysis (Lipponen, 1995). Low level *MYC* (8q) copy gains as detected by fluorescence in situ hybridization were significantly associated with tumour grade, stage and tumour proliferation. There was no association of low level *MYC* copy number increase with high-expression of MYC protein, suggesting it may be a marker for gain of other distal 8q genes (Sauter *et al*, 1995a).

JUN

The *JUN* proto-oncogene has a pivotal role in the regulation of cell proliferation and is involved in signal transduction. Induction of *JUN* causes increased binding to DNA of the transcription factor AP1. JUN oncoprotein immunoreactivity has been detected in the majority of TCCs of the urinary bladder, but there was a significant correlation of increased JUN oncoprotein staining with muscle invasion and EGFR positivity (Tiniakos *et al*, 1994).

EPIDERMAL GROWTH FACTOR RECEPTOR FAMILY

Epidermal Growth Factor Receptor

Epidermal growth factor (EGF) is a 53 aminoacid peptide of 6000 daltons that is found in many tissues. Large quantities are secreted from the submaxillary gland and are also found in milk, urine and prostatic secretions (Kasselberg *et al*, 1985). In vitro studies have shown that growth and division of human cell lines derived from TCC was stimulated by EGF (Messing *et al*, 1984). Thus the presence of corresponding receptors on tumour cells may be important with regard to proliferation. The EGF receptor is the product of the *ERBB1* gene (located on chromosome 17q) and is found in the plasma membrane of many cells. It is a 175 kDa glycosylated transmembrane protein and together with the ERBB2, ERBB3 and ERBB4 gene products belongs to the class 1 growth factor receptors, which are tyrosine kinase receptors (Yarden and Ulrich, 1988). They consist of transmembrane proteins characterized by extracellular binding domains that interact with various growth factors, a hydrophobic region that spans the plasma membrane and an intracellular domain with tyrosine kinase activity. The EGFR is activated by EGF and the alternative ligand—transforming growth factor α (TGFA). TGFA is upregulated in many tumour types, and in one study of TCC levels were shown to correlate better with EGFR status than with tissue EGF, suggesting that TGFA is the more important ligand (Mellon *et al*, 1996a).

Initial interest in the expression of EGFR in bladder cancer stemmed from the finding that more muscle invasive tumours stained more strongly for EGFR than did superficial tumours. In addition EGFR positivity was more common in poorly differentiated tumours than in moderately differentiated tumours. A later prospective study assessing EGFR status in 101 patients with newly diagnosed bladder cancer found that strong staining for the EGFR was associated with high tumour stage and with death. In patients with superficial tumours, EGFR positivity was associated with multiplicity, time to recurrence, recurrence rate and progression (Neal *et al*, 1990). This study was extended to include a total of 212 patients and in multivariate analysis EGFR was confirmed to be a predictor of survival and stage progression independent of tumour stage and grade. In the high risk group of T_1G_3 bladder cancer EGFR status was found to be 80% sensitive and 93% specific in predicting stage progression (Mellon *et al*, 1995).

EGFR overexpression occurs predominantly by mechanisms other than *EGFR* gene amplification. Southern blot analysis revealed a low frequency (1/31) of *EGFR* gene amplification in bladder tumours (Berger *et al*, 1987). Similarly only one case ($T_{3a}G_3$) from 35 (3%) demonstrated *EGFR* gene amplification when assessed by differential PCR (Gorgoulis *et al*, 1995). EGFR mRNA overexpression has been shown to occur more frequently (36%; 5/14) than amplification (Wood *et al*, 1992). Interference with EGFR–ligand interaction may be of clinical benefit, and preclinical immunotherapy studies using neutralizing antibodies directed at the EGFR receptor have been successful in inhibiting growth in vitro of a range of carcinoma cell lines that overexpress EGFR (Dean *et al*, 1994).

ERBB2

The *ERBB2* gene (also known as *neu* or *HER2*), located on chromosome 17q21, encodes a 185 kDa transmembrane phosphoglycoprotein with significant sequence homology to the EGFR (Yamamoto, 1986). Reported candidate ligands are the neuregulin family (NRG1 and NRG2) (Chang *et al*, 1997; Carraway III *et al*, 1997). The finding that *ERBB2* amplification and overexpression were associated with poor clinical outcome in breast cancer has led to the initiation of studies in bladder cancer. The incidence of gene amplification seems to be greater for *ERBB2* than for *EGFR*. Gorgoulis and co-workers (1995) demonstrated amplification of *ERBB2* in about 11% (4/35) of tumours. In a series of 92 patients with bladder cancer, 26% (24/92) exhibited *ERBB2* gene amplification, with a significant relationship with tumour grade (Orlando *et al*, 1996). ERBB2 protein overexpression was found in 21% (20/95) of patients. There was no correlation between increased staining for ERBB2 and tumour stage, grade, or EGFR status, and only 1 of 24 tumours analysed by Southern blotting had evidence of *ERBB2* amplification (Mellon *et al*, 1996b). This indicates that gene amplification is probably not the primary mechanism for increased protein expression, and the clinical significance of *ERBB2* amplification and expression and use as a prognostic marker in bladder cancer still remain controversial. The current research in this area is centred on studies of hetero-dimerization of receptors and consequently on the analysis of co-expression of the family members of *ERBB2*.

LOSS OF HETEROZYGOSITY STUDIES

Deletions and rearrangements of chromosomes are common in human malignancies. Molecular genetic analyses of bladder cancer have uncovered abnormalities in a number of chromosomes, though these changes were initially detected by cytogenetic methods (Gibas *et al*, 1984). With the development of the Human Genome Mapping Project and the advent of advanced molecular techniques such as restriction fragment length polymorphisms (RFLP), fluorescence in situ hybridization (FISH), PCR and microsatellite analysis the allelotype of a particular type of tumour can be characterized and the pattern of chromosome deletions mapped in fine detail. Mapped polymorphic markers are now able to reveal loss of heterozygosity (LOH) and the pattern of chromosome deletions implied can in turn uncover the location of putative tumour suppressor genes.

Molecular studies have demonstrated deletions involving 9p, 9q or both chromosome arms in approximately 60% of bladder tumours of all grades and stages (Cairns *et al*, 1993). As this genotypic alteration is found in low grade, superficial tumours it represents a candidate for an early or initiating event in bladder TCC. T_a bladder tumours appear to present with predominantly 9q abnormalities, whereas T_1 tumours display both altered 9p and 9q deletion genotypes (Orlow *et al*, 1994). Minimal deletion regions on chromosome 9 appear to define two putative tumour suppressor loci on 9q (9q34 between *D9S61* and *D9S66*, and 9q13–q31) and one on 9p21 (Cairns *et al*, 1994; Habuchi *et al*, 1995). Locus 9p21 harbours genes that encode two cyclin dependent kinase inhibitors CDKN2A (p16) and CDKN2B (p15). LOH at the markers *IFNA* and *D9S171*, which are adjacent to *CDKN2B* and *CDKN2A*, have been detected in 41% and 33%, respectively, of informative cases of bladder tumours. However, this LOH could not identify *CDKN2B* or *CDKN2A* as the definite tumour suppressor gene in this region (Packenham *et al*, 1995). With microsatellite markers, LOH of chromosome 9 was demonstrated in 77% of CIS lesions. A high frequency of homozygous deletion surrounding the *CDKN2A* locus, similar to that encountered in superficial TCC, was also described. Many of the chromosomal alterations displayed by muscle invasive tumours have also been demonstrated in CIS lesions, which is consistent with the aggressive nature of CIS lesions (Rosin *et al*, 1995).

Deletions of chromosome 17 are significantly more common in muscle invasive and poorly differentiated bladder tumours. The likely target gene is *TP53*, located on 17p. The majority of tumours with 17p deletions have mutations in the retained *TP53* locus, leaving cells with only the mutant *TP53* gene (Sidransky *et al*, 1991).

Similarly LOH of chromosome 13q in the region of the retinoblastoma (*RB*) locus has been significantly correlated with muscle invasion (Cairns *et al*, 1991). This has been related to loss of expression of the RB protein detected immuno-histochemically (Xu *et al*, 1993).

Chromosome 11p deletions are present in 40% of bladder tumours and have been demonstrated to be associated with high grade tumours (Olumi *et al*, 1990). RFLP and microsatellite analysis show two distinct regions of deletion on 11p (11p15.1–15.2) and 11q (11q13–23.2). These have been shown to occur individually and concurrently in individual tumours, suggesting the presence of two distinct regions of LOH that may harbour putative tumour suppressor genes (Shaw and Knowles, 1995).

Allelic loss of 18q is present in approximately one third of bladder tumours and is significantly related to muscle invasive disease. The *DCC* (*deleted in colorectal carcinoma*) gene has been suggested to be a potential candidate tumour suppressor gene in TCC associated with 18q deletion (Brewster *et al*, 1994).

Allelic analysis has demonstrated LOH of three discrete regions of 3p (Li *et al*, 1996), of 4p and 4q (Polascik *et al*, 1995) and of two regions of 8p (Takle and Knowles, 1996), all significantly associated with higher tumour grade and stage. Other studies have shown two areas of deletion on 14q to be common in muscle invasive bladder cancer (Chang *et al*, 1995). In contrast, Y chromosome loss determined by FISH was a frequent event in TCCs and was not correlated with tumour grade or stage, suggesting that it may occur early in bladder cancer in males (Sauter *et al*, 1995b).

CELL CYCLE AND RETINOBLASTOMA

Most tumour suppressor genes and oncogenes ultimately have effects on cell cycle control. In a normal cell there is a balance between positive and negative influences on progression through the cell cycle. Malignant cells, however, escape from this tight regulatory control. The cell cycle can be considered to consist of four stages (Fig. 2).

Progress through the cell cycle is mediated by cyclin/cyclin dependent kinase (CDK) complexes. During the G_1 phase D and E type cyclins complex with CDK4/CDK6 and CDK2 respectively. These in turn interact with and phosphorylate the RB protein, which regulates the E2F family of transcription factors and thus cell cycle progression. The hypophosphorylated form of the RB protein acts as a powerful growth inhibitory molecule by binding to and inhibiting the E2F/DP1 transcription factor complexes. A family of cyclin dependent kinase inhibitors (CDKIs) negatively regulate the cell cycle, and these include proteins CDKN1A (also known as p21, WAF1 or CIP1), 1B (p27), 2A (p16), 2B (p15) and 2C (p18). CDN2A and 2B inhibit cyclin D/CDK4,6 complexes and prevent the advance of the cell from G_1 to the S phase (Weinberg, 1996).

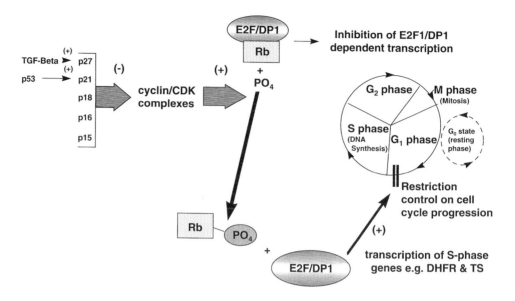

Fig. 2. Cell cycle control. (+) = positive signal (increasing the amount or activity of the target molecule). (−) = negative signal (decreasing the amount or activity of the target molecule). CDK = cyclin dependent kinases. DHFR = dihydrofolate reductase. DP1 = one of the heterodimeric components of E2F. E2F = family of heterodimeric transcriptional regulators. PO_4 = phosphate groups. RB = retinoblastoma protein. TGF-Beta = Transforming growth factor β. TS = thymidylate synthase

CDKN1A inhibits cyclin E/CDK2 and results in hypophosphorylation of RB protein and cell cycle arrest (El Deiry *et al*, 1993).

The *RB* gene, located on chromosome 13q14, was the first tumour suppressor gene isolated (Sparkes *et al*, 1980). It codes for a 110 kDa nuclear phosphoprotein that plays an important part in the cell cycle. Patients who inherit a defective copy of the *RB* gene have a 95% probability of developing bilateral retinoblastoma tumours by the age of seven as a result of inactivation of the remaining normal copy of the gene (Friend *et al*, 1986). Studies of surviving retinoblastoma patients and their relatives have reported a higher than expected incidence of other tumours, including bladder cancer (DerKinderen *et al*, 1988). Evidence now exists that *RB* gene mutation and LOH at 13q are found in sporadic bladder tumours. The RB protein is ubiquitously expressed in normal tissues. Reduced RB expression is shown with immunohistochemical methods to occur in all grades and stages of bladder cancer but is commonly associated with invasive tumours (Presti *et al*, 1991). In addition *RB* gene mutations assessed by PCR and SSCP analysis of RNA have revealed mutations in 21% (4/19) of superficial (pT_a and pT_1) tumours and 36% (4/11) of invasive (pT_2 or greater) tumours (Miyamoto *et al*, 1995). Absence of RB protein expression determined by immunohistochemistry was found in 15 of 17 primary bladder tumours and was associated with LOH at the *RB* locus. Altered RB protein expression was predominantly seen in muscle invasive and high grade tumours (Xu *et al*, 1993). LOH at both the *RB* and the *TP53* loci (see below) in human bladder cancer were found to be associated with muscle invasion ($p<0.05$ and $p<0.025$, respectively). Grade was found to be associated with *TP53* LOH ($p<0.01$) but not with LOH of the *RB* locus. *TP53* LOH and *RB* LOH were often observed simultaneously in some tumours, signifying that these tumour suppressor genes may be interlinked (Miyamoto *et al*, 1996).

Work assessing *MYC* and $TGF\beta_1$ gene (*TGFB1*) expression has revealed no relationship to *RB* gene inactivation (Kubota *et al*, 1995). The presence of mutations of *RB* and *TP53* was found to be associated with recurrence in bladder cancers (Chern *et al*, 1996). When the *RB* gene was introduced into several bladder carcinoma cell lines, inhibition of tumorigenicity was noted, although re-expression of *RB* was not associated with alteration of growth rate in vitro (Goodrich *et al*, 1992). Altered RB expression as assessed by immunohistochemistry has not provided additional prognostic information in terms of patient survival when compared to tumour stage, papillary status or cell proliferation indices, although it may still be an important underlying molecular mechanism (Lipponen and Liukkonen, 1995). Thus current knowledge suggests that RB protein loss is important in invasive tumours and may be related to tumour progression.

TP53 Tumour Suppressor Gene and Bladder Cancer

The *TP53* gene, located on chromosome 17p13.1, has been described as the most commonly altered gene in human cancer. It codes for a 53 kDa stress induced nuclear phosphoprotein, whose main functions are cell cycle arrest, programmed cell death (apoptosis), inhibition of tumour growth, protection against viral infection and preservation of genetic stability. These activities are mediated by transcriptional trans-activation, transcriptional suppression and inhibition of DNA replication (Velculescu and El-Deiry, 1996). TP53 can bind DNA in a sequence specific manner and transcriptionally regulates genes such as *CDKN1A*, *MDM2* (*mouse double minute 2 oncogene homologue*), cyclin G, *BAX* (*BCL2 associated X protein*) and *GADD45* (*growth arrest and DNA damage inducible gene*).

The *TP53* gene is reported to be mutated in over half of all human tumours (Hollstein *et al*, 1991). Inactivation of *TP53* may occur by mutation or deletion of one or both alleles, which can be detected by loss of heterozygosity (LOH) studies. The most common situation appears to be inactivation of one allele by a point mutation, coupled with a deletion of the other allele. Mutation of the *TP53* gene results in the formation of a dysfunctional protein that has a longer half life than the wild type TP53 and accumulates to levels that allow detection by immunohistochemical methods. An association, but not concordance, has been established between TP53 protein overexpression and *TP53* mutations detected by DNA sequencing and SSCP (Vet *et al*, 1995). The presence of TP53 immunoreactivity without *TP53* gene mutations can be attributed to the presence of stabilized forms of the wild type molecule, which may not be in a functionally active state.

Reports have demonstrated higher rates of *TP53* mutations in invasive than in superficial bladder tumours. In a series of 30 patients with superficial bladder tumours the frequency of *TP53* mutations was 13% (4/30)(Yoshimura *et al*, 1995), whereas Spruck and co-workers (1994) reported mutations in 3% (1/36) of superficial tumours and in 51% (25/49) of muscle invasive tumours. In a second study no mutations were found in superficial bladder tumours (0/21), but 33% (8/24) of muscle invasive tumours exhibited mutations, and all mutations were found in grade 3 tumours (Vet *et al*, 1994). In addition the tumours with altered *TP53* showed a higher frequency of allelic loss than the tumours without a mutation, suggesting a correlation between *TP53* mutations and genetic instability. There was also a notable association between poor survival and *TP53* mutations for the whole group. However, *TP53* mutations did not have additional prognostic value in muscle invasive bladder tumours.

The incidence of nuclear TP53 accumulation detected by antibody PAb1801 in patients with CIS was found to be 45% ($\geq$20% tumour cells positive) and was the only independent marker of tumour progression and death in univariate and multivariate analysis (Sarkis *et al*, 1994). The high level of TP53 expression in CIS may explain its propensity to progress.

Immunohistochemical detection of TP53 assessed by the polyclonal antibody CM1 ($\geq$10% nuclear staining) was highly significant in predicting progression in 25 pT_1 bladder tumours, although grade remained the most statistically significant predictor of progression (Thomas *et al*, 1993). However, a similar study utilizing three primary antibodies (CM1, PAb1801 and DO-7) did not find that TP53 immunoreactivity was correlated with outcome (Gardiner *et al*, 1994). These studies highlight the discrepancies of TP53 immunoreactivity in superficial disease: standardized studies need to be conducted for these discrepancies to be resolved. In a series of 243 patients treated with radical cystectomy TP53 immunoreactivity using the monoclonal antibody PAb1801 was significantly associated with an increased risk of recurrence and decreased survival. In this study a multivariate analysis showed nuclear TP53 status to be a predictor of recurrence and survival, independent of stage, grade and lymph node status in cancer confined to the bladder (Esrig *et al*, 1994). In contrast patients with TCC treated with radical cystectomy and adjuvant chemotherapy had significantly fewer recurrences and increased survival if their tumours had altered TP53 as determined immunohistochemically. Correspondingly for patients without TP53 immunoreactivity, adjuvant chemotherapy conferred no benefit in terms of recurrence or survival (Cote *et al*, 1997). These results demonstrate that TP53 status may be able to identify patients with unfavourable bladder tumours and those who would benefit from chemotherapy.

TP53 gene mutations have been demonstrated in urine from bladder cancer patients (Sidransky *et al*, 1991) and in patients with multiple tumours, in all but one of whom the *TP53* mutation was identical to that of the primary tumour. Similarly cells from urine samples from patients with primary bladder cancers demonstrated identical mutations to the tumour itself. In 8 patients in whom a total of 30 urine samples were taken at follow-up cystoscopic examination, 6 of the 24 samples in which mutations were detected were associated with negative cystoscopies. This demonstrates the monoclonal origin of recurrent TCC and the presence of tumour cell clones in urine in the absence of macroscopic evidence of TCC (Xu *et al*, 1996). This theory is reinforced by the finding of identical *TP53* mutations in concomitant transitional cell carcinomas of the renal pelvis and urinary bladder, but not in normal renal tissue from the same patient (Lunec *et al*, 1992).

CDKN1A and *TP53*

TP53 triggers transcription of the *CDKN1A* gene located on chromosome 6p21.2. *CDKN1A* provides a molecular link from *TP53* to control of the cell cycle and is a downstream mediator of TP53 dependent cell cycle checkpoint control. The CDKN1A product inhibits cyclin/CDK phosphorylation of substrates including RB, resulting in inhibition of cell cycle progression at the G_1/S checkpoint. A recent study from Newcastle on a series of 173 patients with primary bladder cancer has demonstrated CDKN1A immunoreactivity to be inversely correlated to tumour stage, grade, TP53 accumulation and Ki67 expression, these relationships being statistically significant. Tumour progression, progression free interval and tumour recurrence were not significantly related to *CDKN1A* positivity in superficial disease. However, CDKN1A positivity in patients with muscle invasive disease was significantly correlated with survival (Braithwaite *et al*, 1997).

MDM2 and *TP53*

The *MDM2* oncogene codes for a 90 kDa nuclear protein, which inhibits TP53 function by concealing the activation domain of TP53 from the cellular transcription machinery (Oliner *et al*, 1993). It has also been demonstrated that TP53 activates the transcription of *MDM2*, which in turn suppresses TP53 function, producing a feedback inhibition regulatory loop that prevents overactivity of TP53 and in particular preventing the triggering of apoptosis by TP53 (Wu *et al*, 1993). *MDM2* may also possess additional oncogenic mechanisms unrelated to *TP53* or *RB* (Sigalas *et al*, 1996).

Highly elevated MDM2 immunoreactivity (monoclonal antibody 2A10) has been reported in 30% (26/87) of bladder tumours, but only one case showed *MDM2* gene amplification. There was a significant association between MDM2 and TP53 overexpression. In addition there was a strong relationship between

MDM2 overexpression and low stage, low grade bladder tumours (Lianes *et al*, 1994). These results suggest a role for *MDM2* in low stage, low grade bladder tumours and possibly a synergistic role with *TP53*.

BCL2, BAX and *TP53* Mediated Apoptosis

Apoptosis is a mechanism of programmed cell death that is important in normal development and in the turnover of cells in regenerating normal adult tissues. It has been suggested that at least one TP53 mediated apoptotic pathway is regulated by the transcription of BAX. BCL2 is a 26 kDa proto-oncogene protein product, which suppresses signals that induce apoptotic cell death (Reed, 1995). BAX, a 21kDa pro-apoptotic protein with 21% homology to BCL2, inhibits the function of BCL2 by forming dimers with it. Loss of apoptotic function in tumour cells may be linked to tumour progression and resistance to chemotherapy and radiotherapy (Arends and Wyllie, 1991). Wild type TP53 stimulates BAX synthesis, which promotes apoptosis by the formation of BCL2-BAX heterodimers and antagonism at BCL2 targets.

In one study BCL2 immunoreactivity (monoclonal BCL2 antibody; Dako, Denmark) was significantly elevated in poorly differentiated bladder tumours (King *et al*, 1996). However, another group, using similar techniques, demonstrated BCL2 immunoreactivity (monoclonal BCL2, clone 124: Dako, USA) to be inversely related to grade and TP53 immunoreactivity (Shiina *et al*, 1996). A further study investigated the ratio of *BCL2/BAX* expression evaluated at the RNA level through a semiquantitative PCR based reaction in bladder tumours (stage $\leq T_{2a}$). A molecular pattern characterized by a *BCL2/BAX* ratio less than one correlated with a significantly higher relapse free time (mean follow-up 17 months) compared with patients with higher levels of *BCL2* than *BAX*.. The *BCL2/BAX* ratio was found to be useful as a marker of recurrence in low grade bladder tumours, independently of stage and grade (Gazzaniga *et al*, 1996).

METALLOPROTEINASES

Degradation of the extracellular matrix (ECM) is an essential process for cancer cells to metastasize. Of particular importance for tumours of epithelial origin is invasion through the basement membrane, consisting of type IV collagen. Metalloproteinases (MMPs) are a family of zinc dependent endopeptidases with proteolytic activity for components of the ECM. Two MMPs in particular have high type IV collagenolytic activity compared with other members of the MMP family, namely MMP2 and MMP9 (Liotta *et al*, 1991). These are regulated by tissue inhibitors of MMPs (TIMPs) by forming an irreversible stoichiometric complex with the activated enzyme and therefore maintaining homoeostasis.

Quantitative zymography has shown MMP9 levels to be significantly higher in bladder tumours than in control samples. There was a significant association between elevated levels of MMP9 and active MMP2 in poorly differentiated tumours. In addition levels were markedly higher in invasive tumours than in superficial disease (Davies *et al*, 1993). In one study serum TIMP1 levels were positively correlated with invasion and metastasis in bladder cancer patients (Naruo *et al*, 1994), and another study found strong correlation between TIMP2 immunoreactivity, loss of basement membrane and poor survival in patients with invasive bladder cancer (Grignon *et al*, 1996). In a series of 53 patients with urothelial cancer with muscular invasion or with lymph node metastasis who underwent complete resection, the ratio of serum MMP2 to TIMP2 was measured. With reference to recurrence and disease free survival, patients with elevated serum MMP2/TIMP2 ratios were of significantly unfavourable status compared with patients with normal values (Gohji *et al*, 1996). MMP1 production and extracellular secretion assessed by northern analysis and enzyme linked immunosorbent assay have been demonstrated to be stimulated by EGF in RT112 bladder tumour cell lines. In addition MMP1 levels have been detectable in urine of patients with bladder tumours, and this may be important in EGFR positive tumours and may relate to outcome (Nutt and Lunec, 1997). Thus the available evidence indicates MMPs and TIMPs are important in bladder cancer, although this needs to be more precisely defined.

ANGIOGENESIS

Angiogensis (neovascularization) is important for continuing tumour growth, progression and metastasis. The process is essential for the progression of a small cluster of abnormal cells to a large metastatic tumour. Without the assistance of angiogenesis to sequester and develop a blood supply, tumours would not become larger than a few millimetres (Folkman, 1996).

Initial studies on angiogenesis have concentrated on quantitative pathology. In a series of 45 muscle invasive bladder tumours using transurethrally resected specimens, microvessel density was assessed using an antibody to the platelet endothelial cell adhesion molecule, CD31. This was demonstrated to be a significant prognostic indicator and to be as informative as stage in predicting overall survival (Dickinson *et al*, 1994). Blood vessel density was confirmed to be significantly correlated with tumour stage and the presence of vascular invasion and was a significant predictor of death from bladder cancer (Philp *et al*, 1996). Similarly immunostaining of endothelial cells for factor VIII related antigen demonstrated a significant correlation between microvessel count in primary bladder tumour cystectomy specimens (stage $\geq T_1$) and the presence of occult lymph node metastasis (Jaeger *et al*, 1995).

The degree of angiogenesis depends on stimulatory and inhibitory factors that are either expressed by the ECM, by the actual tumour or in some circumstances by recruited cells (macrophages). Angiogenic factors have been found in the urine of bladder cancer patients. Elevated levels of basic fibroblast growth factor (FGF2) in urine was found in bladder cancer patients, although these have also been found in other conditions (Nguyen *et al*, 1993). Similarly acidic FGF (FGF1) has been detected in urine of bladder cancer patients and suggested as a potential marker for use as a follow-up tool in non-invasive bladder cancer, although a small proportion of patients with prostate cancer demonstrated FGF1 immunoreactivity in the urine, which would be a complicating factor (Chopin *et al*, 1993). Vascular endothelial growth factor (VEGF) and platelet derived endothelial growth factor (PDEGF) are both regarded as angiogenic. The expression of PDEGF was found to be significantly higher in muscle invasive tumours than in superficial tumours and normal bladder urothelium, but expression of VEGF was significantly higher in superficial tumours than in muscle invasive tumours and normal bladder. In addition VEGF expression was notably higher in superficial tumours (pT_1, G_1/G_2) that recurred at three months than in those that did not recur. Both these angiogenic pathways may be related to tumorigenesis in the bladder (O'Brien *et al*, 1995). The same group demonstrated that elevated expression of midkine (another angiogenic factor) was associated with a poor outcome in muscle invasive bladder cancers, although the number of cases examined was small (O'Brien *et al*, 1996).

A relationship between TP53 expression and angiogenesis has also been implicated. It has been postulated that wild type TP53 inhibits angiogenesis by stimulating the expression of thrombospondin 1 (TSP1), which is a potent inhibitor of angiogenesis (Dameron *et al*, 1994). Similarly wild type TP53 has been shown to down-regulate endogenous VEGF, whereas mutant TP53 has no effect (Mukhopadhyay *et al*, 1995). Reduced immunoreactivity for TSP1 in patients who had undergone radical cystectomy for invasive TCC of the bladder was shown to be an independent predictor of disease recurrence, implying that TSP1 may possess tumour suppressor function by inhibiting angiogenesis (Grossfeld *et al*, 1996). The relative importance of these various angiogenic factors in bladder cancer remains to be fully elucidated.

CELL ADHESION MOLECULES

The metastatic potential of a tumour is partly dependent on the ability of cancer cells to detach. This initial step involves breaking the normal integrity of cell–cell adhesion in tissues. There are at least four families of cell adhesion molecules (immunoglobulin, integrin, selectin and cadherin families). E-cadherin, a 120 kDa transmembrane glycoprotein involved in homotypic calcium dependent intercellular adhesion, has been implicated in a variety of tumours in the maintenance of epithelial integrity. Its function depends on intracellular catenins (α, β and γ), which form a bridge between the cytoplasmic tail of E-cadherin and the actin based cytoskeleton (Nagafuchi and Takeichi, 1988).

In vitro studies have shown the presence of immunoreactivity of E-cadherin in non-invasive bladder carcinoma cell lines RT4 and RT112 compared with invasive cell lines (such as EJ24) that do not express E-cadherin (Frixen *et al*,

1991). A similar relationship has been described in in vivo studies. An immuno-histochemical study revealed that decreased E-cadherin expression in snap frozen tumours was significantly correlated with both increased grade and stage. In addition reduced levels of E-cadherin expression was associated with a decreased three year survival. More importantly this was shown to be significant within the group of patients with muscle invasive disease, indicating that the prognostic value of E-cadherin does not solely reflect the correlation with stage (Bringuier *et al*, 1993). A significantly higher five year survival rate was found in those with preserved membranous E-cadherin staining than in those with decreased staining (Syrigos *et al*, 1995). Reduced levels of E-cadherin expression function have been proposed to occur by alteration of E-cadherin transcriptional regulation, as described in thyroid, squamous cell and colorectal malignancies (Giroldi *et al*, 1995). The autocrine motility factor receptor (gp78) has been shown to be related to E-cadherin. A reduction in E-cadherin with concomitant increase in gp78 expression was found to define a group of patients with bladder cancer with significantly poorer prognosis, though the mechanism of this relationship was unclear (Otto *et al*, 1994).

Soluble forms of E-cadherin have been demonstrated in the circulation of healthy individuals and patients with bladder cancer (Banks *et al*, 1995). Soluble serum E-cadherin (sE-cadherin) concentrations were significantly higher in patients with bladder cancer than in healthy controls. Elevated levels of sE-cadherin significantly correlated to poor histological grade, number of superficial tumours at presentation and a positive three month check cystoscopy in superficial TCC. In addition patients defined as having the lowest risk of recurrence as described by Palmer *et al* (1989) had a median sE-cadherin significantly lower at presentation than the remainder (Griffiths *et al*, 1996). The soluble forms of E-cadherin demonstrated in the serum and urine are probably degradation products of intact E-cadherin found on the urinary tract epithelium and thus may be related to turnover of the molecule. Recently the role of catenins has also been explored in bladder tumours. Decreased expression of E-cadherin, α-, β- and γ-catenins and p120^{cas} (member of the β-catenin/plakoglobin family) was significantly correlated with tumour grade, stage, and poor survival. Proportional hazard regression analysis demonstrated that β-catenin, E-cadherin and α-catenin have similar significant prognostic values. However, in muscle invasive disease only E-cadherin expression had prognostic value (Shimazui *et al*, 1996).

SUMMARY

A large number of potential molecular markers of bladder cancer have been identified, although only a few are truly independent prognostic factors. A number of markers may need to be measured in a single tumour and used as a combination for use in the diagnosis and prognosis of transitional cell carcinoma (TCC).

Epidermal growth factor receptor immunoreactivity has been shown to be an independent predictor of survival and stage progression. TP53 may be an independent predictor of recurrence and overall survival in TCC confined to the bladder, and TP53 alterations may predict chemosensitivity in patients who have had TCC treated by radical cystectomy.

At present molecular techniques such as fluorescence in situ hybridization and the polymerase chain reaction are restricted to the laboratory, but immunohistochemical methods are available in most hospital pathology departments. There are some discrepancies and conflicting reports of the usefulness of molecular markers in different studies, and these need to be addressed in large, prospective, multi-institutional studies using standardized molecular techniques.

References

Arends MJ and Wyllie AH (1991) Apoptosis: mechanisms and roles in pathology. *International Review of Experimental Pathology* **32** 223–254

Banks RE, Porter WH, Whelan P, Smith PH and Selby PJ (1995) Soluble forms of the adhesion molecule E-cadherin in urine. *Journal of Clinical Pathology* **48** 179–180

Berger MS, Greenfield C, Gullick WJ *et al* (1987) Evaluation of epidermal growth factor receptors in bladder tumours. *British Journal of Cancer* **56** 533–537

Braithwaite KL, Mellon JK, Neal DE *et al* (1997) WAF1 expression in transitional cell carcinoma (TCC) of the bladder: inverse relationship to *p53* accumulation and association with good prognosis. *Proceedings of the American Association for Cancer Research* Abstract no. 3534

Brewster SF, Gingell JC, Browne S and Brown KW (1994) Loss of heterozygosity on chromosome 18q is associated with muscle-invasive transitional cell carcinoma of the bladder. *British Journal of Cancer* **70** 697–700

Bringuier PP, Umbas R, Schaafsma E, Karthaus HFM, Debruyne FMJ and Schalken JA (1993) Decreased E-cadherin immunoreactivity correlates with poor survival in patients with bladder tumours. *Cancer Research* **53** 3241–3245

Burchill SA, Neal DE and Lunec J (1994) Frequency of H-*ras* mutations in human bladder cancer detected by direct sequencing. *British Journal of Urology* **73** 516–521

Cairns P, Proctor AJ and Knowles MA (1991) Loss of heterozygosity at the *Rb* locus is frequent and correlates with muscle invasion in bladder carcinoma. *Oncogene* **6** 2305–2309

Cairns P, Shaw ME and Knowles MA (1993) Initiation of bladder cancer may involve deletion of a tumour-suppressor gene on chromosome 9. *Oncogene* **8** 1083–1085

Cairns P, Tokino K, Eby Y and Sidransky D (1994) Homozygous deletion of 9p21 in primary human bladder tumours detected by comparative multiplex polymerase chain reaction. *Cancer Research* **54** 1422–1424

Carraway III KL, Weber JL, Uriger MJ *et al* (1997) Neuregulin-2, a new ligand of ErbB3/ErbB4-receptor tyrosine kinases. *Nature* **387** 512–516

Chang WY, Cairns P, Schoenberg MP, Polascik TJ and Sidransky D (1995) Novel suppressor loci on chromosome 14q in primary bladder cancer. *Cancer Research* **55** 3246–3249

Chang H, Riese II DJ, Gilbert W, Stern DF and McMahan UJ (1997) Ligands for ErbB-family receptors encoded by a neuregulin-like gene. *Nature* **387** 509–512

Chern HD, Becich MJ, Persad RA *et al* (1996) Clonal analysis of human recurrent superficial bladder cancer by immunohistochemistry of *p53* and retinoblastoma proteins. *Journal of Urology* **156** 1846–1849

Chopin DK, Caruelle JP, Colombel M *et al* (1993) Increased immunodetection of acidic fibroblast growth factor in bladder cancer, detectable in urine. *Journal of Urology* **150** 1126–1130

Cote RJ, Esrig D, Groshen S, Jones PA and Skinner DG (1997) *p53* and treatment of bladder cancer. *Nature* **385** 123–125

Dameron KM, Volpert OV, Tainsky MA and Bouck N (1994) Control of angiogenesis in fibroblasts by *p53* regulation of thrombospondin-1. *Science* **265** 1582–1584

Davies B, Waxman J, Wasan H *et al* (1993) Levels of matrix metalloproteinases in bladder cancer correlate with tumour grade and invasion. *Cancer Research* **53** 53 5365–5369

Dean C, Modjtahedi H, Eccles S, Box G and Styles J (1994) Immunotherapy with antibodies to the EGF receptor. *International Journal of Cancer* **Supplement 8** 103–107

DerKinderen DJ, Koten JW, Nagel Kerke NJD *et al* (1988) Non-ocular cancer in patients with hereditary retinoblastoma and their relatives. *International Journal of Cancer* **41** 499–504

Dickinson AJ, Fox SB, Persad RA, Hollyer J, Sibley GNA and Harris AL (1994) Quantification of angiogenesis as an independent predictor of prognosis in invasive bladder carcinomas. *British Journal of Urology* **74** 762–766

El Deiry WS, Tokino T, Velculescu VE *et al* (1993) WAF 1, a potential mediator of *p53* tumour suppression. *Cell* **75** 817–825

Esrig D, Elmajian D, Groshen S *et al* (1994) Accumulation of nuclear *p53* and tumour progression in bladder cancer. *New England Journal of Medicine* **331** 1259–1264

Fitzgerald JM, Ramchurren N, Rieger K *et al* (1995) Identification of H-*ras* mutations in urine sediments complements cytology in the detection of bladder tumours. *Journal of the National Cancer Institute* **87** 129–133

Folkman J (1996) Therapies of the future: fighting cancer by attacking its blood supply. *Scientific American* **275** 116–119

Friend SH, Bernards R, Rogelj *et al* (1986) A human DNA segment with properties of the gene that predisposes to retinoblastoma and osteosarcoma. *Nature* **323** 643–646

Frixen UH, Behrens J, Sachs M *et al* (1991) E-cadherin-mediated cell–cell adhesion prevents invasiveness of human carcinoma cell lines. *Journal of Cellular Biology* **113** 173–185

Gardiner RA, Walsh MD, Allen V *et al* (1994) Immunohistological expression of *p53* in primary pT1 transitional cell bladder cancer in relation to tumour progression. *British Journal of Urology* **73** 526–532

Gazzaniga P, Gradilone A, Vercillo R *et al* (1996) *Bcl-2/bax* mRNA expression ratio as a prognostic marker in low-grade urinary bladder cancer. *International Journal of Cancer (Predictive Oncology)* **69** 100–104

Gibas Z, Prout GR, Connolly JG, Pontis JE and Sandberg AA (1984) Nonrandom chromosomal changes in transitional cell carcinoma of the bladder. *Cancer Research* **44** 1257–1264

Giroldi LA, Bringuier PP and Schalken JA (1995) Defective E-cadherin function in urological cancers: clinical implications and molecular mechanisms. *Invasion and Metastasis* **14** 71–81

Gohji K, Fujimoto N, Fujii A, Komiyama T, Okawa J and Nakajima M (1996) Prognostic significance of circulating matrix metalloproteinase-2 to tissue inhibitor of metalloproteinase-2 ratio in recurrence of urothelial cancer after complete resection. *Cancer Research* **56** 3196–3198

Goodrich DW, Chen Y, Scully P *et al* (1992) Expression of the retinoblastoma gene product in bladder carcinoma cells associates with a low frequency of tumour formation. *Cancer Research* **52** 1968–1973

Gorgoulis VG, Barbatis C, Poulias I and Karameris M (1995) Molecular and immunohistochemical evaluation of epidermal growth factor receptor and ERBB2 gene product in transitional cell carcinomas of the urinary bladder: a study in Greek patients. *Modern Pathology* **8** 758–764

Griffiths TRL, Brotherick I, Bishop RI *et al* (1996) Cell adhesion molecules in bladder cancer: soluble serum E-cadherin correlates with predictors of recurrence. *British Journal of Cancer* **74** 579–584

Grignon DJ, Sakr W, Toth M *et al* (1996) High levels of tissue inhibitor of metalloproteinase-2 (TIMP-2) expression are associated with poor outcome in invasive bladder cancer. *Cancer Research* **56** 1654–1659

Grossfeld GD, Ginberg DA, Stein JP *et al* (1996) Thrombospondin-1 expression as an independent prognostic indicator in invasive transitional cell carcinoma of the bladder. *Proceedings of the American Urological Association* **155** 1508 [Abstract]

Habuchi T, Devlin J, Elder PA and Knowles MA (1995) Detailed deletion mapping of chromosome 9q in bladder cancer: evidence for two tumour suppressor loci. *Oncogene* **11** 1671–1674

Hollstein M, Sidransky D, Vogelstein B and Harris CC (1991) *p53* mutations in human cancers. *Science* **253** 49–53

Jaeger TM, Weidner N, Chew K *et al* (1995) Tumour angiogenesis correlates with lymph node metastasis in invasive bladder cancer. *Journal of Urology* **154** 69–71

Kasselberg AG, Orth DN, Gray ME and Stahlman MT (1985) Immunocytochemical localisation of human epidermal growth factor/urogastrone in several human tissues. *Journal of Histochemical Cytochemistry* **33** 315–322

Kern WH (1984) The grade and pathological stage of bladder cancer. *Cancer* **53** 1185–1189

King ED, Matteson J, Jacobs SC and Kyprianou N (1996) Incidence of apoptosis, cell proliferation in transitional cell carcinoma of the bladder: association with tumour progression. *Journal of Urology* **155** 316–320

Knowles MA and Williamson M (1995) Mutation of H-*ras* is infrequent in bladder cancer: confirmation by single-strand conformation polymorphism, designed restriction fragment length polymorphism, and direct sequencing. *Cancer Research* **53** 133–139

Kotake T, Saiki S, Kinouchi T, Shiku H and Nakayama E (1990) Detection of c-*myc* gene product in urinary bladder cancer. *Japanese Journal of Cancer Research* **81** 1198–1201

Kubota Y, Miyamoto H, Noguchi S *et al* (1995) The loss of retinoblastoma gene in association with c-*myc* and transforming growth factor-β1 gene expression in human bladder cancer. *Journal of Urology* **154** 371–374

Li M, Zhang ZF, Reuter VE and Cordon-Cardo C (1996) Chromosome 3 allelic losses and microsatellite alterations in transitional cell carcinoma of the urinary bladder. *American Journal of Pathology* **149** 229–235

Lianes P, Orlow I, Zhang Z *et al* (1994) Altered patterns of MDM2 and *p53* expression in human bladder cancer. *Journal of the National Cancer Institute* **86** 1325–1330

Liebert M and Seigne J (1996) Characteristics of invasive bladder cancers: histological and molecular markers. *Seminars in Urologic Oncology* **14** 62–72

Liotta LA, Steeg PS and Stetler-Stevenson WG (1991) Cancer metastasis and angiogenesis: an imbalance of positive and negative regulation. *Cell* **64** 327–336

Lipponen PK (1995) Expression of c-*myc* protein is related to cell proliferation and expression of growth factor receptors in transitional cell bladder cancer. *Journal of Pathology* **175** 203–210

Lipponen PK and Liukkonen TJ (1995) Reduced expression of retinoblastoma gene protein is related to cell proliferation and prognosis in transitional-cell bladder cancer. *Journal of Cancer Research and Clinical Oncology* **121** 44–50

Lunec J, Challen C, Wright C, Mellon K and Neal DE (1992) c-*erb*B-2 amplification and identical p53 mutations in concomitant transitional carcinomas of renal pelvis and urinary bladder. *Lancet* **339** 439–440

Mellon JK, Wright C, Kelly P, Horne CHW and Neal DE (1995) Long-term outcome related to epidermal growth factor receptor status in bladder cancer. *Journal of Urology* **153** 919–925

Mellon JK, Cook S, Chambers P and Neal DE (1996a) Transforming growth factor-α levels in bladder cancer and their relationship to epidermal growth factor receptor. *British Journal of Cancer* **73** 654–658

Mellon JK, Lunec J, Wright C, Horne CHW, Kelly P and Neal DE (1996b) *ERBB2* in bladder cancer: molecular biology, correlation with epidermal growth factor receptors and prognostic value. *Journal of Urology* **155** 321–326

Messing EM, Bubbers JE, Dekernion JB and Fahey JL (1984) Growth stimulating activity produced by human bladder cancer cells. *Journal of Urology* **132** 1230–1234

Miyamato H, Shuin T, Torigoe S *et al* (1995) Retinoblastoma gene mutations in primary human bladder cancer. *British Journal of Cancer* **71** 831–835

Miyamoto H, Shuin T, Ikeda I *et al* (1996) Loss of heterozygosity at the *p53*, *Rb*, DCC and *APC* tumour suppressor gene loci in human bladder cancer. *Journal of Urology* **155** 1444–1447

Mostofi FK, Sobin LH and Torlini H (1973) *Histological Typing of Urinary Bladder Tumours*, World Health Organization, Geneva

Mukhopadhyay D, Tsiokas L and Sukhatme VP (1995) Wild-type *p53* and *v-Src* exert opposing influences on human vascular endothelial growth factor gene expression. *Cancer Research* **55** 6161–6165

Nagafuchi A and Takeichi M (1988) Cell binding function of E-cadherin is regulated by the cytoplasmic domain. *Journal of European Membrane Biology* **7** 3679–3684

Narayana AS, Loening SA, Slymen DJ and Culp DA (1983) Bladder cancer: factors affecting survival. *Journal of Urology* **130** 56–60

Naruo S, Kanayama H, Takigawa H, Kagawa S, Yamashita K and Hayakawa T (1994) Serum levels of a tissue inhibitor of metalloproteinases-1(TIMP-1) in bladder cancer patients. *International Journal of Urology* **1** 228–231

Neal DE, Sharples L, Smith K, Fennelly J, Hall RR and Harris AL (1990) The epidermal growth factor receptor and the prognosis of bladder cancer. *Cancer* **65** 1619–1625

Nguyen M, Watanabe H, Budson AE, Richie JP and Folkman J (1993) Elevated levels of the angiogenic peptide basic fibroblast growth factor in urine of bladder cancer patients. *Journal of the National Cancer Institute* **85** 241–242

Nutt J and Lunec J (1997) Production of matrix metalloproteinase 1 (MMP1) by bladder tumour cells following EGF stimulation. *Proceedings of the British Association of Cancer Research* Abstract No 2.1

O'Brien T, Cranston D, Fuggle S, Bicknell R and Harris A (1995) Different angiogenic pathways characterise superficial and invasive bladder cancer. *Cancer Research* **55** 510–513

O'Brien T, Cranston D, Fuggle S, Bicknell R and Harris A (1996) The angiogenic factor midkine is expressed in bladder cancer, and overexpression correlates with a poor outcome in patients with invasive cancers. *Cancer Research* **56** 2515–2518

Oliner JD, Pietenpol JA, Thiagalingam S, Gyuris J, Kinzler KW and Vogelstein B (1993) Oncoprotein *MDM2* conceals the activation domain of tumour suppressor *p53*. *Nature* **362** 857–860

Olumi AF, Tsai YC, Nichols PW *et al* (1990) Allelic loss of chromosome 17p distinguishes high grade from low grade transitional cell carcinomas of the bladder. *Cancer Research* **50** 7081–7083

Orlando C, Sestini R, Vona G *et al* (1996) Detection of ERBB2 amplification in transitional cell bladder carcinoma using competitive PCR technique. *Journal of Urology* **156** 2089–2093

Orlow I, Lianes P, Lacombe L, Dalbagni G, Reuter VE and Cordon-Cardo C (1994) Chromosome 9 allelic losses and microsatellite alterations in human bladder tumours. *Cancer Research* **54** 2848–2851

Otto T, Birchmeier W, Schmidt U *et al* (1994) Inverse relation of E-cadherin and autocrine motility factor receptor expression as a prognostic factor in patients with bladder carcinomas. *Cancer Research* **54** 3120–3123

Packenham JP, Taylor JA, Anna CH, White CM and Devereux TR (1995) Homozygous deletions but no sequence mutations in coding regions of *p15* or *p16* in human primary bladder tumours. *Molecular Carcinogenesis* **14** 147–151

Palmer MKB, Freedman LS, Hargreave TB and Tolley DA (1989) Prognostic factors for recurrence and follow-up policies in the treatment of superficial bladder cancer: report from the British medical research council subgroup on superficial bladder cancer (Urological cancer working party). *Journal of Urology* **142** 284–287

Philp EA, Stephenson TJ and Reed MWR (1996) Prognostic significance of angiogenesis in transitional cell carcinoma of the human urinary bladder. *British Journal of Urology* **77** 352–357

Polascik TJ, Cairns P, Chang WYH, Schoenberg MP and Sidransky D (1995) Distinct regions of allelic loss on chromosome 4 in human primary bladder carcinoma. *Cancer Research* **55** 5396–5399

Presti JC, Reuter VE, Galan T *et al* (1991) Molecular genetic alterations in superficial and locally advanced human bladder cancer. *Cancer Research* **51** 5405–5409

Rosin MP, Cairns P, Epstein JI, Schoenberg MP and Sidransky D (1995) Partial allelotype of carcinoma in-situ of the human bladder. *Cancer Research* **55** 5213–5216

Sarkis AS, Dalbagni G, Cordon-Cardo C *et al* (1994) Association of *p53* nuclear over-expression and tumour progression in carcinoma in situ of the bladder. *Journal of Urology* **152** 388–392

Sauter G, Carroll P, Moch H *et al* (1995a) c-*myc* copy number gains in bladder cancer detected by fluorescence in-situ hybridization. *American Journal of Pathology* **146** 1131–1139

Sauter G, Moch H, Wagner U *et al* (1995b) Y chromosome loss detected by FISH in bladder cancer. *Cancer Genetics and Cytogenetics* **82** 163–169

Shaw ME and Knowles MA (1995) Deletion mapping of chromosome 11 in carcinoma of the bladder. *Genes, Chromosomes and Cancer* **13** 1–8

Shiina H, Igawa M, Urakami S, Honda S, Shirakawa H and Ishibe T (1996) Immunohistochemical analysis of *bcl-2* expression in transitional cell carcinoma of the bladder. *Journal of Clinical Pathology* **49** 395–399

Shimazui T, Schalken JA, Giroldi LA *et al* (1996) Prognostic value of cadherin-associated molecules (α-,β–, and γ-catenins and p120^{cas}) in bladder tumours. *Cancer Research* **56** 4154–4158

Sidransky D, Eschenbach AV, Tsai YC *et al* (1991) Identification of *p53* gene mutations in bladder cancers and urine samples. *Science* **252** 706–709

Sigalas I, Calvert AH, Anderson JJ, Neal DE and Lunec J (1996) Alternatively spliced *MDM2* transcripts with loss of *p53* binding domain sequences: transforming ability and frequent detection in human cancer. *Nature Medicine* **2** 912–917

Sparkes RS, Sparkes MC, Wilson MG *et al* (1980) Regional assignment of genes for human esterase D and retinoblastoma to chromosome band 13q14. *Science* **208** 1042–1044

Spruck CHR, Ohneseit PF, Gonzalez-Zulueta M *et al* (1994) Two molecular pathways to transitional cell carcinoma of the bladder. *Cancer Research* **54** 784–788

Syrigos KN, Krausz T, Waxman J *et al* (1995) E-cadherin expression in bladder cancer using formalin-fixed, paraffin-embedded tissues: correlation with histopathological grade, tumour stage and survival. *International Journal of Cancer (Predictive Oncology)* **64** 367–370

Takle LA and Knowles MA (1996) Deletion mapping implicates two tumour suppressor genes on chromosome 8p in the development of bladder cancer. *Oncogene* **12** 1083–1087

Thomas DJ, Robinson MC, Charlton R, Wilkinson S, Shenton BK and Neal DE (1993) *p53* expression, ploidy and progression in pT1 transitional cell carcinoma of the bladder. *British Journal of Urology* **73** 533–537

Tiniakos DG, Mellon K, Anderson JJ, Robinson MC, Neal DE and Horne CHW (1994) c-*jun* oncogene expression in transitional cell carcinoma of the urinary bladder. *British Journal of Urology* **74** 757–761

Velculescu VE and El-Deiry WS (1996) Biological and clinical importance of the *p53* tumour suppressor gene. *Clinical Chemistry* **42:6** 858–868

Vet JAM, Bringuier PP, Poddighe PJ, Karthaus HFM, Debruyne FMJ and Schalken JA (1994) *p53* mutations have no additional prognostic value over stage in bladder cancer. *British Journal of Cancer* **70** 496–500

Vet JAM, Bringuier PP, Schaafsma HE, Witjes JA, Debruyne MJ and Schalken JA (1995) Comparison of *p53* protein overexpression with *p53* mutation in bladder cancer: clinical and biological aspects. *Laboratory Investigation* **73** 837–843

Weinberg RA (1996) How cancer arises. *Scientific American* **275** 32–40

Wood DP Jr, Fair WR and Chaganti RS (1992) Evaluation of epidermal growth factor receptor DNA amplification and mRNA expression in bladder cancer. *Journal of Urology* **147** 274–277

Wu X, Bayle JH, Olson D and Levine AJ (1993) The *p53-MDM2* autoregulatory feedback loop. *Genes and Development* **7** 1126–1132

Xu H, Cairns P, Hu S *et al* (1993) Loss of *Rb* protein expression in primary bladder cancer correlates with loss of heterozygosity at the *Rb* locus and tumour progression. *International Journal of Cancer* **53** 781–784

Xu X, Stower MJ, Reid N, Garner RC and Burns PA (1996) Molecular screening of multifocal transitional cell carcinoma of the bladder using *p53* mutations as biomarkers. *Clinical Cancer Research* **2** 1795–1800

Yamamoto T, Ikawa S, Akiyama T *et al* (1986) Similarity of protein encoded by the human *ERBB2* gene to epidermal growth factor receptor. *Nature* **319** 230–234

Yarden Y and Ulrich A (1988) Growth factor receptor tryosine kinases. *Annual Review of Biochemistry* **57** 443

Yoshimura I, Kudoh J, Saito S, Tazaki H and Shimizu N (1995) *p53* gene mutations in recurrent superficial bladder cancer. *Journal of Urology* **153** 1711–1715

The authors are responsible for the accuracy of the references.

Clinical Evaluation of Immunotherapy: Are There Differences between Papillary and Flat In Situ Bladder Cancer?

DONALD L LAMM

Department of Urology, Robert C Byrd Health Sciences Center of West Virginia University, Morgantown, West Virginia

Introduction
Immunotherapy and chemotherapy differences
Papillary and flat in situ carcinoma differences
Clinical studies of intravesical chemotherapy
Carcinoma in situ
Clinical BCG immunotherapy studies
Summary

INTRODUCTION

Immunotherapy with bacillus Calmette-Guérin (BCG) is universally recognized as the optimal intravesical treatment for transitional cell carcinoma in situ (CIS) of the bladder, but controversy persists regarding the superiority of BCG immunotherapy over intravesical chemotherapy, particularly mitomycin, in the prophylaxis of recurrent papillary tumours. Some hold that if BCG has not been demonstrated to be superior to mitomycin in preventing recurrence of papillary tumours, mitomycin should be the treatment of choice because it has fewer side effects. Is the response to immunotherapy different in CIS and papillary bladder cancer? Is BCG immunotherapy superior to mitomycin chemotherapy in papillary as well as in situ carcinoma? I will review the current clinical data and present my perspective on these important clinical questions.

IMMUNOTHERAPY AND CHEMOTHERAPY DIFFERENCES

To determine whether or not differences exist in the responses of papillary and in situ bladder cancer to immunotherapy versus chemotherapy we should begin with a consideration of the basic differences between immunotherapy and chemotherapy. The mechanism of action of BCG immunotherapy is incompletely defined but is vastly different from that of chemotherapy. Intravesical BCG instillation stimulates a local cellular immune response and an associated release of a wide variety of cytokines such as interleukin 2, tumour necrosis factor and interferon γ (Prescott *et al*, 1989; Bohle *et al*, 1990, 1993; O'Donnell *et al*, 1996). Immune stimulation generally peaks with the sixth instillation in patients who have not been previously treated (DeBoer L, personal communication). In patients who receive a subsequent course of BCG, immune stimulation generally peaks at the third instillation, and continued treatment or excessively high doses of BCG will suppress the immune response (Lamm *et al*, 1982a; Reichert and Lamm, 1984; Ratliff and Catalona, 1989; DeBoer L, personal communication). The immune stimulation that results from BCG instillation persists for many months and results in tumour destruction. Cytotoxic chemotherapy, in contrast, has well defined mechanisms of action such as alkylation (mitomycin, thiotepa, epodyl) or intercalation and topoisomerase II inhibition (doxorubicin). Cell destruction depends on direct contact with the cancer cell and is proportional to drug concentration and duration of exposure (Walker *et al*, 1986). BCG attaches to tumour cells by means of specific receptors (fibronectin and integrin) (Ratliff, 1994) and can penetrate deep into the bladder wall and be carried to regional lymph nodes and beyond. Chemotherapeutic drugs are non-specific and penetrate the bladder by concentration gradient diffusion. The deepest tumour cells—those that are most likely to give rise to recurrence and progression—therefore unfortunately receive the least effective drug treatment.

With completely different mechanisms of action it might be expected that immunotherapy and cytotoxic chemotherapy produce different responses in papillary and in situ bladder cancer. The onset of action of chemotherapy is quick: the drugs can be retained for only about 2 hours, and little remains after voiding. The onset of action of BCG is slow: 6 weeks are required for optimum stimulation of the immune response, and it sometimes takes 6 months for immune destruction to be complete. The "prophylactic" effect of intravesical chemotherapy depends on destruction of occult malignancy or transformed cells, because chemotherapy is active at the time of administration. In contrast, BCG can induce immune stimulation that persists and can potentially destroy new tumours as they start to emerge. Immediate instillation of chemotherapy following tumour resection could be expected to reduce seeding and directly inhibit tumour growth, but BCG has no direct activity on tumour cells, and immediate instillation has proven to be highly toxic (Rawls *et al*, 1990). The configuration of CIS would potentially increase the efficacy of either treatment, as would papillary configuration and absence of invasion compared with solid configuration, decreased vascularity or invasion. Finally, biological differences such as the multiple drug resistance phenotype or tumour antigenicity could make individual tumours resistant to one mode of therapy but sensitive to another.

PAPILLARY AND FLAT IN SITU CARCINOMA DIFFERENCES

Carcinoma in situ is recognized as a highly variable but generally aggressive malignancy that has high potential to invade and metastasize. Even in grade 3, stage T_1 tumours the concomitant presence of CIS appears to increase the risk of disease progression significantly (Vicente *et al*, 1991; Holmang *et al*, 1997). Superficial papillary transitional cell carcinoma is perhaps even more variable. ranging from nearly innocuous to potentially lethal. In a review of six reported series only 5% of patients with grade 1, stage T_a tumours had progression when followed for an average of 9 years, compared with 38% of patients with grade 3, stage T_1 tumours followed for an average of less than 5 years (Bostwick, 1992). The erroneous conclusion that grade 1 tumours are not a threat to the patient must be avoided: of all patients who progressed to muscle invasive disease, 25% initially had grade 1, stage T_a or T_1 carcinoma (Bostwick, 1992).

The obvious differences between papillary and in situ bladder cancer would be expected to result in different sensitivities to immunotherapy and chemotherapy. Certainly individual malignancies will respond to one agent and not the other, but regrettably we currently are unable to predict such responses. Are there generalities that can be made? Is the superiority of response to BCG immunotherapy limited to CIS, high grade or lamina propria invasive carcinomas? To answer these questions we will review the reported clinical studies.

CLINICAL STUDIES OF INTRAVESICAL CHEMOTHERAPY

Table 1 lists the results of 26 chemotherapy trials that enrolled 4739 patients in randomized comparisons of surgery alone versus surgery plus intravesical chemotherapy. Overall, 14 of these 26 studies reported statistically significant reduction in tumour recurrence with intravesical chemotherapy. A total of 1257 patients enrolled in 11 controlled thiotepa studies, 6 of which achieved statistical significance (Lamm *et al*, 1995b). The relative advantage of thiotepa versus surgery alone averaged 15%. The most significant reduction in tumour recurrence occurred in the 2 studies (Burnand *et al*, 1976; Zincke *et al*, 1983) that used a single early postoperative thiotepa instillation. If we eliminate the large Medical Research Council (MRC) 1985 study that used a dilute concentration of thiotepa, 30 mg in 60 ml, from the trials listed in Table 1, the relative benefit of thiotepa increases to a level that is at least as high as that of the commonly used newer chemotherapies. A total of 1446 patients enrolled in 6 doxorubicin controlled studies, 3 of which achieved statistical significance. As in the thiotepa studies, the greatest benefit of doxorubicin was noted when a single early postoperative treatment was given. Zincke *et al* (1983) noted a 39% reduction in tumour recurrence with a single 50 mg doxorubicin instillation. Overall, the relative advantage of doxorubicin treatment versus surgery alone was a 16% reduction in tumour recurrence. A total of 1329 patients enrolled in 6 randomized controlled mitomycin C trials, 3 of which achieved statistical significance. Overall, tumour recurrence was reduced by an average of 10% with mitomycin. Ethoglucid resulted in a 31% reduction in tumour recurrence in a European Organization for Research on Treatment of Cancer (EORTC) study, and in 2 epirubicin studies tumour reduction averaged 11%.

TABLE 1. Effect of intravesical chemotherapy on recurrence in controlled studies of patients undergoing transurethral resection of bladder tumour

Reference	No of patients	No with recurrence (%)		Difference % with recurrence	p value*
		Treated	**Controls**		
THIOTEPA					
Burnand et al, 1976	51	31 (97)	11 (58)	39	0.001
Byar & Blackard, 1977	86	29 (60)	18 (47)	13	0.016
Nocks et al, 1979	42	14 (64)	13 (65)	−1	NS
Asahi et al, 1980	134	23 (41)	31 (40)	1	NS
Schulman et al, 1982	209	72 (69)	62 (59)	10	NS
Koontz et al, 1981	93	31 (66)	18 (39)	27	0.02
Zincke et al, 1983	58	20 (71)	9 (30)	41	0.002
Prout et al, 1983	90	43 (76)	29 (64)	12	0.05
Medical Research Council, 1985	367	46 (37)	97 (40)	−3	NS
Netto and Lemos, 1983	34	16 (80)	6 (43)	37	NS
Hirao et al, 1992	93	22 (46)	7 (15)	31	0.0015
Total	1257	338 (59)	301 (44)	15 (advantage)	
DOXORUBICIN					
Niijima et al, 1983	436	86 (62)	135 (45)	17	0.05
Zincke et al, 1983	59	20 (71)	10 (32)	39	0.01
Kurth et al, 1985	217	41 (59)	52 (35)	24	0.006
Rubben et al, 1988	220	50 (61)	77 (56)	5	NS
Akaza et al, 1987	457	49 (33)	77 (25)	8	NS
Abrams et al, 1981	57	25 (89)	23 (79)	10	NS
Total	1446	271 (55)	374 (39)	16 (NS)	
MITOMYCIN C					
Huland et al, 1984	79	16 (52)	5 (10)	42	0.01
Niijima et al, 1983	278	86 (62)	79 (57)	5	NS
Kim & Lee, 1989	43	18 (82)	17 (81)	1	NS
Tolley et al, 1988	397	85 (65)	137 (51)	14	0.001
Krege et al, 1996	234	56 (46)	30 (27)	19	0.004
Akaza et al, 1987	298	49 (33)	36 (24)	9	NS
Total	1329	310 (52)	304 (41)	11 (NS)	
ETHOGLUCID					
Kurth et al, 1985	209	41 (59)	39 (28)	31 (advantage)	0.0004
EPIRUBICIN					
Oosterlinck et al, 1993	399	84 (41)	56 (29)	12	0.0152
Melekos, 1993	99	19 (59)	27 (40)	19	NS
Total	498	103 (43)	83 (32)	11	
Cumulative Result	4739	1063 (54)	1101 (40)	14 (advantage)	

*p value as reported by the authors

NS = not significant

Advantage is defined as the total % recurrence following transurethral resection alone minus % recurrence following surgery plus intravesical chemotherapy. Lengths of follow-up and risk factors vary from study to study, so statistical comparisons, other than those reported by original authors, are not appropriate and are not reported. Averages are presented for interest only

From these controlled chemotherapy trials we can conclude that: (a) chemotherapy clearly reduces tumour recurrence, (b) the reduction in tumour recurrence ranges from –3 to 42% (average 14%), (c) there is no evidence that the newer and more costly chemotherapies are superior to the older treatments (thiotepa or ethoglucid), and (d) an early single postoperative instillation of an appropriate concentration of chemotherapy appears to offer protection that is as good if not better than more extensive delayed treatments.

In most studies the observed reduction in tumour recurrence was limited to 2–3 years, but the meta-analysis of 2535 patients entered into EORTC and MRC studies followed for 7.7 years confirmed a long term statistically significant reduction of 7% (Pawinski *et al*, 1996). Unfortunately, as has been confirmed by extensive literature review (Lamm, 1992b), there was no evidence to suggest that reduction in tumour recurrence with chemotherapy is associated with a reduction in tumour progression.

CARCINOMA IN SITU

In the treatment of CIS the reported overall complete response is 48% in 448 patients treated with chemotherapy—38% in 89 patients treated with thiotepa, 48% in 212 patients treated with doxorubicin and 53% in 147 patients treated with mitomycin (Lamm, 1992b). Controlled chemotherapy trials provide no evidence that any of the newer chemotherapies provides superior protection from tumour recurrence, but in the historical CIS studies above comparisons show a statistically significantly higher complete response rate with mitomycin than with thiotepa. There is no statistically significant advantage of mitomycin over doxorubicin. Currently more than 1500 patients with CIS have been treated with BCG, and the overall complete response proportion is 72% (Lamm, 1995). The complete response rate is statistically significantly higher with BCG immunotherapy than with mitomycin, doxorubicin or thiotepa. More importantly, whereas in most series fewer than 20% of patients treated with chemotherapy remain disease free for 5 years, 64% of patients with complete response to BCG remain disease free when treated with suboptimal treatment schedules (Lamm *et al*, 1991). With maintenance BCG schedules using instillations each week for 3 weeks at 3 months, 6 months and every 6 months to 3 years, the estimated 5 year disease free rate is 75% (Lamm, 1992a).

CLINICAL BCG IMMUNOTHERAPY STUDIES

Controlled comparisons of BCG immunotherapy versus surgery alone have demonstrated statistically significant reduction in tumour recurrence in each of 6 studies (Herr *et al*, 1985, 1986; Lamm, 1985; Pagano *et al*, 1991; Melekos *et al*, 1993; Krege *et al*, 1996). The reduction in tumour recurrence has ranged from 20 to 65% and averages 38% (Table 2). These consistent statistically significant results and the more than doubled improvement in the advantage of

TABLE 2. Effect of intravesical BCG on recurrence in controlled studies

Reference	No of patients	CONTROL (TURBT)		BACILLUS CALMETTE-GUÉRIN			
		Controls	No with recurrence (%)	Treated	No with recurrence (%)	Difference % recurrence	p value
Lamm, 1985	57	27	14 (52)	30	6 (20)	32	<0.001
Herr *et al*, 1985	86	43	41 (95)	43	18 (42)	53	<0.001
Herr *et al*, 1986	49	26	26 (100)	23	8 (35)	65	<0.001
Pagano *et al*, 1991	133	63	52 (83)	70	18 (26)	57	<0.001
Melekos *et al*, 1993	94	32	19 (59)	62	20 (32)	27	<0.02
Krege *et al*, 1996	224	122	56 (46)	102	26 (26)	20	0.003
Total	643	313	208 (67)	330	96 (29)	38	

immunotherapy, each compared with surgery alone, suggests that BCG provides superior prophylaxis for recurrent papillary transitional cell carcinoma as well as superior treatment for CIS.

As illustrated in Table 3, direct randomized comparisons of BCG and chemotherapy prophylaxis show a consistent statistically significant advantage of BCG over thiotepa (3 of 3 studies) and doxorubicin (2 of 2 studies), but the advantage of BCG over mitomycin has been inconsistent (3 of 6 studies). This latter inconsistency is fully compatible with the expected results of clinical trials in bladder cancer and does not mean, as has been stated elsewhere, that "mitomycin is equal to BCG in the prophylaxis of T_a, T_1 bladder cancer." We need only remember that 3 of 6 controlled mitomycin trials showed no significant advantage of mitomycin therapy over surgery alone, and that does not mean that "mitomycin is shown to be no better than surgery alone."

Controlled trials have failed to show an advantage of mitomycin over other intravesical chemotherapies, but the complete response of CIS to mitomycin is historically higher than that to thiotepa. Failure to show a statistically significant advantage does not, of course, mean that no advantage exists. The studies done often had insufficient power and could have detected only major differences between groups.

TABLE 3. Overview of controlled trials of BCG vs chemotherapy for superficial bladder cancer[a]

	Median rate of recurrence, BCG arm	Median rate of recurrence, chemotherapy arm	No of positive trials
BCG vs thiotepa	7%	42%	3/3
BCG vs doxorubicin	38%	64%	2/2
BCG vs mitomycin	30%	43%	3/6

[a]Summarized from Lamm and Torti (1996)

It has been suggested for both thiotepa and mitomycin C that responses are more frequent in lower grade tumours. With BCG immunotherapy our experience is that high grade tumours may be more responsive (Lamm *et al*, 1982b). The inclusion of a high percentage of low grade tumours may also explain the failure of 3 of the previous 6 studies to demonstrate the superiority of BCG over mitomycin C. In the Southwest Oncology Group comparison of BCG and mitomycin, with 378 evaluable patients, overall tumour recurrence was reduced from 55% in patients randomized to mitomycin C to 42% in patients receiving BCG (Lamm *et al*, 1995). Tumour recurrences tended to be of lower grade in the BCG arm and of higher grade in the mitomycin C arm: only 4 grade III or anaplastic tumours occurred in the BCG arm, compared with 12 such recurrences in the mitomycin C arm.

The Southwest Oncology Group comparison of a single 6 week course and maintenance with BCG using 3 weekly instillations at 3, 6, 12, 18, 24, 30 and 36 months provides further evidence that the advantage of BCG over chemotherapy is not primarily limited to patients with CIS (Lamm *et al*, 1990, 1997). In all previous studies patients with CIS responded best to BCG, but in the maintenance study the advantage of BCG was greatest in patients with recurrent T_a, T_1 transitional cell carcinoma. This observation suggests that, as documented from animal studies decades ago (Bast *et al*, 1974), optimal immune response to BCG occurs when the organism is given in direct juxtaposition to tumour cells. With papillary tumours, transurethral resection may frequently remove all cancer cells, whereas with CIS complete resection is rare. Therefore, the previously reported increased sensitivity of CIS to BCG immunotherapy appears to be related to the technique of administration rather than an intrinsic sensitivity.

SUMMARY

The advantage of BCG immunotherapy over intravesical chemotherapy in superficial bladder cancer has been most apparent in patients with carcinoma in situ (CIS), where complete response is increased from 50% to more than 70% and the proportion of patients remaining disease free for 5 years is increased from 20% to 40%. Similar advantages have been reported using suboptimal BCG treatment schedules in patients with recurrent stage T_a, T_1 tumours. BCG provides long term protection from tumour recurrence and, unlike chemotherapy, reduces tumour progression. The observed relative increased sensitivity of CIS to BCG and the occasional failure of BCG to demonstrate significant superiority over mitomycin C in the prevention of tumour appear to be related to the use of suboptimal BCG treatment schedules. With maintenance BCG using 3 weekly instillations at 6 month intervals, patients with papillary tumours fare even better than patients with CIS, and tumour progression is even further reduced. Chemotherapy is appropriate for patients who are at very low risk of tumour progression and those who fail to respond to BCG, but overall the results of BCG immunotherapy are superior for patients with either CIS or T_a, T_1 transitional cell carcinoma.

References

Abrams PH, Choa RG, Gaches CG, Ashken MH and Green NA (1981) A controlled trial of single dose intravesical adriamycin in superficial bladder tumours. *British Journal of Urology* **53** 585–587

Akaza H, Isaka S, Koiso K *et al* (1987) Comparative analysis of short-term and long-term prophylactic intravesical chemotherapy of superficial bladder cancer. *Cancer Chemotherapy and Pharmacology* **20 (Supplement)** 91–94

Asahi T, Matsumura Y, Tanahashi T *et al* (1980) The effects of intravesical instillation of thiotepa on the recurrence rate of bladder tumors. *Acta Medica Okayama* **34** 43–45

Bast RC Jr, Zbar B, Borsos T *et al* (1974) BCG and cancer, 1. *New England Journal of Medicine* **290** 1413–1415

Bohle A, Nowc Ch, Ulmer AJ *et al* (1990) Detection of urinary TNF, IL1, and IL2 after local BCG immunotherapy for bladder carcinoma. *Cytokine* **2** 175–181

Bohle A, Thanhauser A, Ulmer AJ *et al* (1993) Dissecting the immunobiological effects of bacillus Calmette-Guérin (BCG) in vitro: evidence of a distinct BCG-activated killer (BAK) cell phenomenon. *Journal of Urology* **150** 1032–1034

Bostwick D (1992) Natural history of early bladder cancer. *Journal of Cellular Biochemistry* **161 (Supplement)** 31

Brosman SA (1982) Experience with bacillus Calmette-Guérin in patients with superficial bladder cancer. *Journal of Urology* **128** 27–30

Burnand KG, Boyd PJR, Mayo ME, Shuttleworth KED and Lloyd-Davies RW (1976) Single dose intravesical thiotepa as an adjuvant to cyclodiathermy in the treatment of transitional cell bladder carcinoma. *British Journal of Urology* **48** 55–57

Byar D and Blackard C (1977) Comparisons of placebo, pyridoxine, and topical thiotepa in preventing recurrence of stage I bladder cancer. *Urology* **10** 556–558

Herr HW, Pinsky CM, Whitmore WF, Sogani PG, Oettgen HF and Melamed MR (1985) Experience with intravesical bacillus Calmette-Guérin therapy of superficial bladder tumors. *Urology* **25** 119–121

Herr HW, Pinsky CM, Whitmore WF, Sogani PG, Oettgen HF and Melamed MR (1986) Long-term effect of intravesical bacillus Calmette-Guérin on flat carcinoma in situ of the bladder. *Journal of Urology* **135** 265–268

Hirao Y, Okajima E, Ozono S *et al* (1992) A prospective randomized study of prophylaxis of tumor recurrence following transurethral resection of superficial bladder cancer—intravesical thio-TEPA versus oral UFT. *Cancer Chemotherapy and Pharmacology* **30 (Supplement)** S26–S30

Holmang S, Hedelin H, Anderstrom C, Holmberg E and Johansson SL (1997) The importance of the depth of invasion in T_1 bladder carcinoma: a prospective cohort study. *Journal of Urology* **157** 800–804

Huland H, Otto U, Drose M and Kloppel G (1984) Long-term mitomycin C instillation after transurethral resection of superficial bladder carcinoma: influence on recurrence, progression, and survival. *Journal of Urology* **132** 27–29

Kim HH and Lee C (1989) Intravesical mitomycin C instillation as a prophylactic treatment of superficial bladder tumor. *Journal of Urology* **141** 1337–1340

Koontz WW Jr, Prout GR Jr, Smith W, Frable WJ and Minnis JE (1981) The use of intravesical thio-tepa in the management of non-invasive carcinoma of the bladder. *Journal of Urology* **125** 307–309

Krege S, Giani G, Meyer R *et al* (1996) A randomized multicenter trial of adjuvant therapy in superficial bladder cancer: transurethral resection only versus transurethral resection plus mitomycin versus transurethral resection plus bacillus Calmette-Guérin. *Journal of Urology* **156** 962–966

Kurth KH, Debruyne FJM, Senge T *et al* (1985) Adjuvant chemotherapy of superficial transitional cell carcinoma: an EORTC randomized trial comparing doxorubicin hydrochloride, ethoglucid and TUR alone, In: Schroeder FH and Richards B (eds). *Part B: Superficial*

Bladder Tumors (EORTC Genitourinary Group Monograph 2, part B), pp 135–142, Alan R Liss, New York

Lamm DL (1985) Bacillus Calmette-Guérin immunotherapy for bladder cancer. *Journal of Urology* **134** 40–42

Lamm DL (1992a) Carcinoma in situ. *Urologic Clinics of North America* **19** 499–508

Lamm DL (1992b) Long-term results of intravesical therapy for superficial bladder cancer. *Urologic Clinics of North America* **19** 573–580

Lamm DL (1995) BCG immunotherapy for carcinoma in situ of the bladder. *Oncology* **9** 947–956

Lamm DL, Reichert FD, Harris SC and Lucio RM (1982a) Immunotherapy of murine transitional cell carcinoma. *Journal of Urology* **128** 1104–1108

Lamm DL, Thor DE, Stogdill VD and Radwin HM (1982b) Bladder cancer immunotherapy. *Journal of Urology* **128** 931–935

Lamm DL, Sarosdy MF, Grossman HB *et al* (1990) Maintenance vs. nonmaintenance BCG immunotherapy of superficial bladder cancer: a Southwest Oncology Group study. *Journal of Urology* **143** [Abstract 610, p 341]

Lamm DL, Blumenstein BA and Crawford ED (1991) A randomized trial of intravesical doxorubicin and immunotherapy with bacille Calmette-Guérin for transitional cell carcinoma of the bladder. *New England Journal of Medicine* **325** 1205–1209

Lamm DL, Blumenstein BA and Crawford ED (1995a) Randomized intergroup comparison of bacillus Calmette-Guérin immunotherapy and mitomycin C chemotherapy prophylaxis in superficial transitional cell carcinoma of the bladder: a Southwest Oncology Group study. *Urologic Oncology* **1** 119–126

Lamm DL, Riggs DR, Trayneus CL, and Naeyo ON (1995b) Failure of current intravesical cell carcinomas of the bladder. *Journal of Urology* **53** 1444–1450

Lamm DL and Torti F (1996) Bladder cancer. *Ca - A Cancer Journal for Clinicians* **46** 103–112

Lamm DL, Blumenstein B, Sarosdy MF, Grossman B and Crawford ED (1997) Significant long-term patient benefit with BCG maintenance therapy: a Southwest Oncology Group study. *Journal of Urology* **157** [Abstract 831, p 213]

Malmstrom Lundholm C, Norlen JB and Ekman P *et al* (1996) A randomized prospective study comparing long-term intravesical instillations of mitomycin C and bacillus Calmette-Guérin in patients with superficial bladder carcinoma. *Journal of Urology* **156** 372–376

Medical Research Council (1985) The effect of intravesical thiotepa on the recurrence rate of newly diagnosed superficial bladder cancer. *British Journal of Urology* **57** 680–683

Melekos MD (1993) Prophylaxis of superficial bladder cancer with a modified intravesical epirubicin treatment schedule. *Oncology* **50** 450–455

Melekos MD, Chionis H, Pantazakos A, Fokaefs E, Paranychianakis G and Dauaher H (1993) Intravesical bacillus Calmette-Guérin immunoprophylaxis of superficial bladder cancer: results of a controlled prospective trial with modified treatment schedule. *Journal of Urology* **149** 744–746

Netto NR and Lemos GC (1983) A comparison of treatment methods for the prophylaxis of recurrent superficial bladder tumors. *Journal of Urology* **129** 33–34

Niijima T, Akaza H, Koiso K and the Japanese Urologic Cancer Research Group for Adriamycin (1983) Randomized clinical trial on chemoprophylaxis of recurrence in cases of superficial bladder cancer. *Cancer Chemotherapy* **2 (Supplement)** 579–583

Nocks BN, Nieh PT and Prout GR Jr (1979) A longitudinal study of patients with superficial bladder carcinoma successfully treated with weekly intravesical thiotepa. *Journal of Urology* **122** 27–29

O'Donnell MA, Xiaohong C and DeWolf WC (1996) Maturation of the cytokine immune response to bacillus Calmette-Guérin (BCG) in the bladder: implications for treatment schedules. *Journal of Urology* **155** 568A

Oosterlinck W, Kurth KH, Schrder F *et al* (1993) A prospective European Organization for Research and Treatment of Cancer Genitourinary Group randomized trial comparing transurethral resection followed by a single intravesical instillation of epirubicin or water in single state T_a, T_1 papillary carcinoma of the bladder. *Journal of Urology* **149** 749–752

Pagano F, Bassi P, Milani C, Meneghini A, Maruzzi D and Garbeglio A (1991) A low dose bacillus Calmette-Guérin regimen in superficial bladder cancer therapy: is it effective? *Journal of Urology* **146** 32–35

Pawinski A, Bouffioux C, Sylvester R, Parmar M, Smith P and van der Meijden A for the EORTC-GU group and British MRC (1996) Meta-analysis of EORTC/MRC randomized clinical trials for the prophylactic treatment of T_a, T_1 bladder cancer. *Journal of Urology* **155** 492A [Abstract 727, p 492]

Prescott S, James K, Hargreave TB *et al* (1989) Immunopathological effects of intravesical BCG therapy, In: Debruyne FMJ, Denis L and van der Meijden ADPM (eds). *BCG in Superficial Bladder Cancer* (EORTC Genitourinary Group Monograph 6), pp 93–105, Alan R Liss, New York

Prout GR Jr, Koontz WW Jr, Coombs LJ, Hawkins IR and Friedell GH for the National Bladder Cancer Collaborative Group (1983) Long-term fate of 90 patients with superficial bladder cancer randomly assigned to receive or not to receive thiotepa. *Journal of Urology* **130** 677–680

Ratliff TL (1994) Mechanism of action of intravesical BCG for superficial bladder cancer, In: Pagano F and Bassi P (eds). *BCG Immunotherapy in Bladder Cancer*, pp 25–31, Cooperative Libraria Editrice Universita di Padova, Padova

Ratliff TL and Catalona WJ (1989) Depressed proliferative responses in patients treated with 12 weeks of intravesical BCG. *Journal of Urology* **141** [Abstract 244, p 230]

Rawls WH, Lamm DL, Lowe BA *et al* (1990) Fatal sepsis following intravesical bacillus Calmette-Guérin administration for bladder cancer. *Journal of Urology* **144** 1328–1330

Reichert DF and Lamm DL (1984) Long term protection in bladder cancer following intralesional immunotherapy. *Journal of Urology* **132** 570–573

Rubben H, Lutzeyer W, Fischer N *et al* (1988) Natural history and treatment of low and high risk superficial bladder tumors. *Journal of Urology* **139** 283–285

Schulman CC, Robinson M, Denis L *et al* (1982) Prophylactic chemotherapy of superficial transitional cell bladder carcinoma: an EORTC randomized trial comparing thiotepa, VM-26 and TUR alone. *European Urology* **8** 207–210

Tolley DA, Hargreave TB, Smith PH *et al* (1988) Effect of intravesical mitomycin C on recurrence of newly diagnosed superficial bladder cancer: interim report from the Medical Research Council Subgroup on Superficial Bladder Cancer. *British Medical Journal* **296** 1759–1763

Vicente J, Laguna MP, Duarte D, Algaba F and Chechile G (1991) Carcinoma in situ as a prognostic factor for $G3pT_1$ bladder tumours. *British Journal of Urology* **68** 380–384

Walkes MC, Master JRW, Parris CN *et al* (1986) Intravesical chemotherapy: in vitro studies on the relationship between dose and toxicity. *Virology Research* **14** 137–139

Zincke H, Utz DC, Taylor WF, Myers RP and Leary FJ (1983) Influence of thiotepa and doxorubicin instillation at time of transurethral surgical treatment of bladder cancer on tumor recurrence: a prospective, randomized, double-blind, controlled trial. *Journal of Urology* **129** 505–508

The author is responsible for the accuracy of the references.

Clonal Development of Bladder Cancer and Its Relevance to the Clinical Potential of HLA Antigen and *TP53* Based Gene Therapy

A M E NOURI • R T D OLIVER • V H NARGUND

Departments of Oncology & Urology, QMW School of Medicine & Dentistry, St Bartholomew's and Royal London Hospitals, Smithfield, London EC1A 7BE

Introduction
Clonal development of bladder cancer
    Contribution of cytogenetics and virology to understanding morphology
    Epidemiology and clonal progression
    Autocrine loops and clonal progression
    Markers of clonal progression
        Telomerase
        Angiogenesis
        Metalloproteinases
HLA and adhesion molecule defects in bladder cancer
In vitro and in vivo rationale for HLA class I gene therapy in early bladder cancer
Clinical models to justify combined *TP53* and HLA class I gene therapy in advanced metastatic bladder cancer
    The *TP53* model in germ cell cancer
    Viral oncolysis as an explanation of renal cell cancer spontaneous regression
The potential of combination gene therapy
Summary

INTRODUCTION

It is more than 12 years since the first demonstration in experimental animal models that correction of tumour cell histocompatibility antigen defects by gene therapy was capable of inducing bystander immunity so that animals could resist challenge with untransfected tumour cells (Hui *et al*, 1984). Several authors have since reported that HLA class I and class II losses as well as adhesion molecule losses are frequent events in a variety of human malignancies and in some cases are associated with increasing degrees of malignancy (Vanky *et al*, 1990; Nouri *et al*, 1994; Tomlinson and Bodmer, 1995; Bicknell *et al*, 1996; Browning *et al*, 1996). The most convincing demonstration of the importance of HLA loss in escape from immune surveillance is a study in lymphoma, which demonstrates that when compared to spontaneous tumours the incidence of

HLA loss is substantially less frequent in tumours arising when immune surveillance is weakened by T lymphocyte immune deficiency such as HIV infection or transplantation immunosuppression (List *et al*, 1993).

The aim of this chapter is to consider new views on the heterogeneity of bladder cancers from the study of the genetics and molecular biology of the clonal development and how this impacts on developing gene therapy studies in this tumour. The review will focus particularly on the role of autocrine growth factor loops arising from work on granulocyte-colony stimulating factor (G-CSF) and human chorionic gonadotrophin (hCG) expression in these tumours and the contribution of HLA loss in these tumours to escape from immune surveillance. These observations provide the background for our proposal for HLA-B7 gene therapy in bladder cancer patients who are candidates for salvage cystectomy because of localized recurrences resistant to conventional treatment. Because this has involved gene therapy in patients with a very good chance of longterm cure, albeit with a diminished quality of life, the ethical issues involved have led to some hesitation by the regulatory authorities to approve the study. These issues will be reviewed in addition to the in vitro studies that have been undertaken to provide the rationale for this study, as well as the limited follow-up information from the studies in patients with terminal melanoma, breast and cervical cancer who have been the first to receive this therapy (Nabel *et al*, 1996; Hui *et al*, 1997). This chapter will end with a review of developments of combination gene therapy, in particular the potential of combination HLA and *TP53* gene therapy, that have arisen from the study of response to chemotherapy of germ cell cancer and the study of viral oncolysis in spontaneous regression in patients with metastatic renal cell cancer that have provided possible clues to how gene therapy could be developed for use in patients with widely disseminated metastatic disease with multiple genetic defects.

CLONAL DEVELOPMENT OF BLADDER CANCER

Contribution of Cytogenetics and Virology to Understanding Morphology

It is now 20 years since it was first proposed (Pugh, 1973) that there might be at least two separate lineages in the development of bladder cancer, one starting with papillary non-invasive tumours and evolving to mixed papillary and solid invasive tumours, and the second pathway starting with flat in situ carcinoma, progressing to pure solid carcinoma (Fig. 1). Today, modern cytogenetics may help to understand this better as loss of chromosome 9q is a significant discriminant of early tumours (Spruck *et al*, 1994). The losses of heterozygosity associated with further progression to invasive and metastatic disease are similar to those seen in colon cancer. One of the most important involves chromosome 17 affecting expression of the *TP53* gene, whose importance in determining response to chemotherapy will be discussed in greater detail later in the

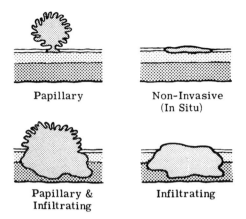

Papillary

Non-Invasive
(In Situ)

Papillary &
Infiltrating

Infiltrating

Fig. 1. Morphological classification of superficial and invasive bladder cancer (Pugh, 1973; reproduced with permission from John Wiley and Sons, Inc)

chapter. The observation from cystoscopy studies that there are variable morphological types of bladder cancer, such as the fine feathered and mulberry types reported by Blandy and England (Fig. 2) raise the question whether there might not be more than two initiating events (Oliver *et al*, 1989a). These observations are the basis for raising the question how many of the multiple variant subtypes of human papillomavirus subtypes (now more than 95; Chan *et al*, 1995) have the ability to initiate spontaneous bladder cancer as has been shown in bladder cancers arising in immunosuppressed individuals (Rovere *et al*, 1988) and those with condyloma acuminata (Wilson *et al*, 1990).

Epidemiology and Clonal Progression

It has long been known that smoking and exposure to industrial chemicals are is associated with excess risk of mortality from bladder cancer (Dolin, 1991). These issues will be examined in greater detail elsewhere in this volume (see Droller). Of particular clinical relevance to understanding the clonal evolution of bladder cancer is that little is known about whether any of these or any other factors influence the progression through the cytogenetic cascade. Smoking is one factor that has emerged from our own work. While much has been done on the role of smoking as an initiation factor in cancer, the evidence that smokers with breast, melanoma and testis cancer have a more malignant variant has been less emphasized as evidence that continued smoking is capable of acting as a promoter of progression through the malignant clonal cascade. In bladder cancer there seem to be two possible mechanisms of action. In the first place, in a small study of patients receiving bacille Calmette-Guérin (BCG) immunotherapy we found a higher relapse rate in smokers compared to non-smokers, which suggests that they had reduced immune resistance (Table 1). Support for this view comes from much larger studies of smoking in patients with early cervical cancer that demonstrated that smoking reduces CD4/CD8

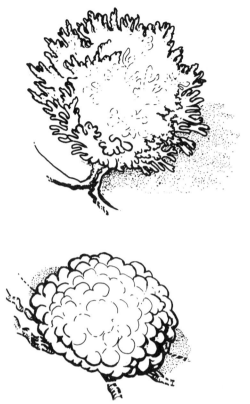

Fig. 2. Diagrammatic representation of extremes of morphological type of papillary carcinoma of the bladder. (Artwork kindly provided by JP Blandy)

ratios and local immune response (Slattery *et al*, 1989). The second study in our patients indicated that persistent heavy smoking in bladder cancer patients may be a factor in accelerated progression to metastasis (Table 2). A report that smoking in bladder cancer is associated with a characteristic mutation of the *TP53* gene (Spruck *et al*, 1993) provides a possible genetic mechanism to explain the association, given the data from loss of heterozygosity showing that chromosome 17 losses are related to late events.

TABLE 1. Influence of smoking on durability of BCG induced complete response (>12 months) in superficial bladder cancer

	No of cases	Proportion with durable complete response at 12 months (%)
Non-smokers with complete response	9	78
Smokers with complete response	6	17
Fisher's exact test: p = 0.041		

TABLE 2. Smoking history and clinical stage of bladder cancer (Oliver, 1989a)

	No of cases	**≥20 cigarettes/day (%)**
Superficial	51	8
Metastatic and invasive	60	25

$\chi^2 = 4.64$, p<0.05

Autocrine Loops and Clonal Progression

There is increasing acceptance of the idea that one component contributing to the clonal evolution of cancer is the development of an autocrine loop whereby the tumour switches on expression of growth factor production and its receptor in the same cell. This idea was first developed in breast cancer to explain escape from hormone dependence (Dickson and Lippman, 1997). There are two observations from our work that suggest that induction of autocrine loops may be a genetic factor that increases the degree of malignancy in bladder cancer. The first is production of G-CSF by the tumour. It is now more than 10 years since the first discovery that bladder cancer cell lines in vitro produce G-CSF (Ito et al, 1990). More recently Japanese workers have provided evidence that these same tumour cells express a receptor for G-CSF (Ohigashi et al, 1992), suggesting that under certain circumstances G-CSF may be acting as an autocrine growth factor in this tumour. Clinical evidence that G-CSF production by bladder cancer is of greater importance than previously suspected comes from a study which correlated the level of circulating granulocyte at time of diagnosis with outcome after radiation. As the level of granulocytosis was the most significant prognostic factor in a multivariate analysis (Daruwalla P et al, unpublished), this prognostic factor analysis provides the first evidence that a G-CSF autocrine loop may be playing a significant part in vivo. Interestingly, this risk factor was synergistic with the degree of lymphopenia in predicting a poor prognosis, which suggests that immune surveillance may be an additive factor.

The second possible autocrine growth factor loop discovered from work in our unit that might be involved in the clonal progression of bladder cancer is the production of a truncated core form of βhCG (Iles et al, 1990; Lazar et al, 1995). hCG is a normal pregnancy associated trophoblast product, and there is some speculation that it may act on the epithelial growth factor receptor whose expression has been demonstrated by several studies to be associated with a poor prognosis in bladder cancer (Neal et al, 1985). Our observations (Oliver et al, 1989c) arose because of a patient who, after nearly 10 years of multiple recurrent superficial cancer, presented with fulminating lung and liver metastases and was dead in 6 weeks. Because he had gynaecomastia his blood was tested and his hCG level was found to be in excess of 1 million IU compared to a normal value of less than 50 IU. Studies also demonstrated that detectable hCG was predominantly present in patients with metastases and that these patients did very badly when treated with chemotherapy (Oliver *et al*, 1989c). The finding that hCG expression was synergistic with squamous metaplasia in predicting poor prognosis (Martin *et al*, 1989) provided additional justification for the study of human papillomavirus expression, as they are most characteristically associated with squamous tumours of cervix and skin.

Markers of Clonal Progression

Telomerase

Telomerase activity has recently been described in many types of malignant tumours including bladder carcinoma (Yoshida *et al*, 1997). Telomerase is a ribonucleoprotein that can compensate for the loss of DNA sequence at the end of each chromosome that occurs at each cell division (Morin, 1989). The telomerase activity is seen in embryonic cells and adult stem cells. However, it is reactivated in cancer cells, suggesting that this enzyme may be important in the proliferation of tumour cells (Rhyu, 1995). Work by one of us (VN) has demonstrated that the telomerase activity can be detected in bladder cancer regardless of stage and differentiation in 85% of the patients studied but is more pronounced in early stages (Nargund *et al*, 1996). Similar results have been described in superficial bladder cancer by Kamata *et al* (1996). Modulation of telomerase and its gene could be used as a treatment in dysplastic lesions and in early stages of bladder cancer.

Angiogenesis

There is now evidence to show that in various malignancies including bladder cancer (Folkmann, 1990) tumour growth is dependent on induction of angiogenesis in order to expand beyond the 2 mm diameter module, which, because of oxygen, glucose and CO_2 diffusion rates, is the maximum size a tumour nodule can grow without developing a new blood supply. Various components, involving endothelial cells, tumour cells, tumour infiltrating cells and extracellular matrix, probably contribute to angiogenesis (Folkman and Shing, 1992). The induction of angiogenesis occurs as a result of substances released from extracellular matrix and tumour cells (Folkman and Shing, 1992). Although the exact cascade is not clear, there are at least two separate angiogenic molecules (vascular endothelial growth factor in superficial bladder cancer and platelet derived endothelial growth factor in invasive bladder cancer) involved at different stages of bladder cancer development (O'Brien *et al*, 1995). Because various studies have demonstrated that a high level of vascular density is associated with a poor prognosis (O'Brien *et al*, 1995; Jaeger *et al*, 1995), targeting the molecules regulating angiogenesis could lead to new treatment approaches to control the progression of bladder cancer.

Metalloproteinases

The degradation of basement membrane by type IV collagenases and other proteases has been suggested as the second step in bladder cancer clonal progression after induction of angiogenesis because these enzymes facilitate the early steps in invasion and metastasis (Liotta, 1986). As the levels of matrix metalloproteinase expression correlates with bladder tumour grade and invasion (Davies *et al*, 1993), it is likely that they are involved in this stage of bladder cancer clonal progression.

HLA AND ADHESION MOLECULE DEFECTS IN BLADDER CANCER

Normal trophoblast lacks HLA and this is thought to be a factor in the escape from immune surveillance of the semiallogeneic trophoblast in utero. This knowledge led us to investigate the role of histocompatibility antigen loss (HLA major histocompatibility complex, MHC) in bladder cancer as a factor in its escape from immune surveillance and as an explanation for the poor survival of βhCG positive tumours (Oliver *et al*, 1989c; Nouri *et al*, 1991, 1992). Snap frozen tissue from 92 patients has been examined. Although total loss of monomorphic HLA antigen expression as defined by monoclonal antibody W6/32 positivity is rare, variable degrees of polymorphic and free heavy chain loss are more frequent (Table 3) and, as a consequence, few tumours do not have some degree of loss. Most interesting is the observation that loss of HLA-B locus antigen appears to occur more frequently than HLA-A locus loss. As it has long been known that HLA-B locus incompatibility produces more frequent rejection than HLA-A locus in kidney transplant recipients (Oliver, 1976), the relative antigenic "strength" of this locus in terms of rejection power could explain why B locus antigen loss is more frequent in tumours than loss of A locus antigen. Substantially larger series will however be needed to prove that this difference is truly an effect of the relative importance of the HLA A and B loci rather than the specific effect of certain alleles as has been suggested by other authors (Tomlinson and Bodmer, 1995).

As the only correlation between HLA expression and clinical behaviour in bladder cancer is an apparent association between HLA antigen loss and occurrence of the G3 poor risk bladder tumours (Table 4), more clinicopathological correlative studies are needed.

A measure of the increasing complexity of cell membrane antigen alterations that support the idea that stepwise clonal evolution does occur in bladder cancer is the observation that in addition to HLA class I loss, there are also cases with altered expression of HLA class II as well as intercellular adhesion molecule 1 (ICAM1) and leucocyte function associated antigen 3 expression. As the norm is for class II and ICAM1 not to be expressed, their expression is an indication of inflammatory exudate cytokine induction. In studies of immunotherapy the expression of class II has been associated with a good prognosis. Our own data have not yet been fully analysed in respect of this, though it is already clear

TABLE 3. Monomorphic and polymorphic HLA-A and B locus class I antigens on bladder tumours

	Negative (%)	Intermediate or strong positive (%)
Monomorphic		
HLA-A, B, C (n=92)	8	24 + 68
β_2-m (n=60)	7	38 + 55
heavy chain (n=57)	38	41 + 21
Polymorphic		
HLA-A locus		
A2 (n=26)	11	39 + 42
A3 (n=10)	10	40 + 50
HLA-B locus		
B7 (n=7)	57	42 + 0
Bw4 (n=26)	38	57 + 4
Bw6 (n=34)	14	59 + 27

from a 2 x 2 comparison of class II and ICAM1 expression (Table 5) that there is a degree of heterogeneity in behaviour that might have clinical significance.

A further measure of the heterogeneity of potential escape mechanisms of bladder cancer comes from studying the response of tumour cell line MHC antigens to γ interferon. These studies illustrate that as well as both relative and absolute resistance to upregulation of HLA class I in some cell lines, others have lost the ability to respond to γ interferon by upregulation of HLA class II (Nouri *et al*, 1992).

IN VITRO AND IN VIVO RATIONALE FOR HLA CLASS I GENE THERAPY IN EARLY BLADDER CANCER

Several animal models (Itaya *et al*, 1987; Hui *et al*, 1989; Clements *et al*, 1992) have demonstrated the principle that correction of major histocompatibility antigen defect leads to the ability to induce bystander immune resistance to

TABLE 4. Correlation of grade and monomorphic HLA class I antigen losses in bladder cancer

	No of cases	Strong positive (%)	Intermediate positive (%)	Complete negative (%)
G1	19	74	15	11
G2	39	74	16	10
G3	13	46	31	23

TABLE 5. Correlation between HLA class I and ICAM1 expression in bladder cancer biopsy specimens

	Class II	
ICAM1	**Positive**	**Negative**
Positive	12	3
Negative	13	21

uncorrected tumour cells. When HLA antigen is re-expressed in deficient tumour cells they are capable of processing antigens and expressing peptides (Toshitani *et al*, 1996). Furthermore, at least two groups (Nabel *et al*, 1996; Hui *et al*, 1997) have demonstrated that intratumoral injection of a liposomal allogeneic HLA class I antigen gene is associated with augmented cytolytic T lymphocyte response in about two thirds and localized tumour rejection in more than one third of patients with melanoma, breast and cervical cancer treated in these studies (Table 6), and in one of these studies there was anecdotal evidence of bystander rejection of uninjected tumour (Nabel *et al*, 1996). The critical issue is whether the evidence of HLA loss in bladder cancer is sufficient to justify such studies in that tumour and in which cases. A further critical issue for all these studies is whether the therapy should be aiming to restore self HLA to normal or is any allogeneic HLA class I antigen sufficient. The lack of a reproducible assay to measure cytolytic T lymphocyte response is one factor slowing progress in this respect.

It is clear from what has been presented in the previous section that in terminal metastatic and poor risk cases the accumulation of multiple genetic defects makes an approach to monogene therapy unrealistic for these patients. It was this realization that led us to focus on using liposomal HLA-B7 gene therapy in patients with multiply recurrent superficial and early invasive bladder cancer who, having failed conventional therapy, were candidates for salvage cystectomy, because even with modern bladder reconstruction (Lerner and Skinner, 1996) these patients suffer some reduction in quality of life. The other advantage of this model is that the tumours are easily accessible for repeated

TABLE 6. Gene therapy studies in cancer

	No of cases	No of responses (CR + PR)	No of curable responses >12 months
HLA-B7 in melanoma (Nabel *et al*, 1996)	14	1 + 6	3
HLA-A2 in ovary/cervix/lung (Hui *et al*, 1997)	8	3 + 3	Nil
HLA-B13 (Hui *et al*, 1997)	6	0 + 1	Nil
TP53 in hepatoma (Fricker, 1996)	8	1 + 3	2
TP53 in lung cancer (Roth *et al*, 1996)	7	2 + 1	Nil
Total	43	7 + 14 (49%)	5 (12%)

CR = complete response; PR = partial response

inspection using flexible cystoscopy, which does not require an anaesthetic, and tumours could be repeatedly injected. A final advantage of this study is that were the HLA-B7 gene therapy study to be positive, it would open up a completely new approach for all cases with superficial bladder cancer as there is some cytogenetic evidence that the current approach using transurethral electrodiathermy may actually be implanting tumour cells in the bladder wall and contributing to the frequency and extent of tumour recurrence (Weldon and Soloway, 1975; Soloway and Masters, 1980).

Figure 3 summarizes our protocol, which is currently being prepared for submission to the Gene Therapy Advisory Committee. The idea of genome altering therapy being used in patients with a condition that is not life threatening and in whom there are still no good laboratory parameters for monitoring specific anti-tumour immune responses has led to some delay in getting approval. This delay has given us time to explore aspects of the study in vitro. The first issue has been whether gene therapy should reconstitute self MHC or whether allogeneic class I is adequate. Although the Zinkernagel and Doherty (1979) studies of viral mediated cytotoxic T lymphocyte (CTL) induction would suggest that self MHC is critical for effective CTL response, there are in vitro immunotherapy experiments with acute myeloid leukaemia that suggest that allo HLA may be very effective in inducing self restricted CTL, particularly if mixed directly with self tumour cells (Zarling *et al*, 1976; Lee and Oliver, 1978; Oliver and Lee, 1978). What is not clear, however, is whether, given the large number of different class I antigens (at least 350 at 13 different loci), all degrees of allo HLA incompatibilities are equally effective for inducing helper response against self restricted tumour antigens. Given that the data suggesting that loss of HLA-B locus is more frequent than loss of HLA-A locus in tumours mirrors information from transplantation on possible differential antigenic strength, it is possible that information from studying the role of the so called "long" HLA-B locus inclusion antigens, W4/W6, could make selection of the appropriate gene easier. These B locus inclusion antigens demonstrated almost as much influence on transplant rejection as would be achieved by matching for the low frequency polymorphics (Table 7). These results suggested that there may be only a limited number of alleles that need to be mismatched to produce maximum immune stimulatory help. Clearly, however, examination of these concepts using in vitro models will be required to be sure. Our own studies so far have been limited. Before deciding on using the allogeneic HLA-B7 gene we considered using the β_2-microglobulin gene for the minority who have complete loss of HLA due to a β_2-microglobulin gene defect in order to enable re-expression of self HLA. Though we were able to demonstrate re-expression of HLA class I in one cell line with such a defect (Nouri *et al*, 1994), it was soon obvious that the relative rarity of such cases (Table 3) made it an unrealistic protocol to pursue for clinical trials. Subsequently, we have compared a complete retroviral plasmid based HLA-B7 with naked HLA-B7 DNA in a cationic liposome and found no advantage for the former. Though we were able to demon-

Screening
cystoscopy:

Pre-study period 1ˢᵗ
TUR

Intratumoral
injection of 250 µg
DNA every
week x 3

Follow-up

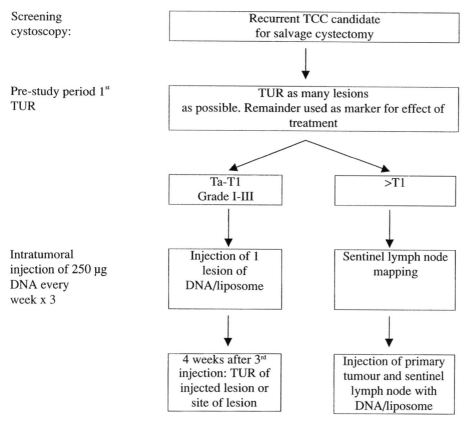

| Recurrent TCC candidate for salvage cystectomy |

| TUR as many lesions as possible. Remainder used as marker for effect of treatment |

Ta-T1 Grade I-III   >T1

Injection of 1 lesion of DNA/liposome   Sentinel lymph node mapping

4 weeks after 3ʳᵈ injection: TUR of injected lesion or site of lesion   Injection of primary tumour and sentinel lymph node with DNA/liposome

1. Follow-up of CR until recurrence or up to study month 25, every 3 months
2. Treatment failure will proceed to cystectomy

Fig. 3. Outline proposal for HLA-B7 gene therapy in bladder patients who are candidates for salvage cystectomy. TCC = transitional cell carcinoma; TUR = transurethral resection; CR = complete response

strate that correcting the HLA defect did reduce NK self non-specific cytotoxicity (Nouri *et al*, 1992), so far we have been unable to devise a specific T cell cytotoxic assay and this remains our immediate priority before starting the pro-

TABLE 7. HLA matching and renal graft survival at 12 months (modified from Oliver, 1976)

	Totally matched (%)	50% matched (%)	Totally incompatible (%)
Total HLA-A locus matching	46% (n = 92)	46% (n = 200)	42% (n = 30)
A locus inclusion matching	45% (n = 61)	44% (n = 64)	44% (n = 53)
Total HLA-B locus matching	63% (n = 61)	49% (n = 189)	42% (n = 72)
B locus inclusion matching	58% (n = 68)	44% (n = 128)	39% (n = 68)

tocol. The recent demonstration of interleukin 2 (IL2) activation in peripheral blood after BCG (Kaempfer *et al*, 1996) gives some clues for developing such an assay.

CLINICAL MODELS TO JUSTIFY COMBINED *TP53* AND HLA CLASS I GENE THERAPY IN ADVANCED METASTATIC BLADDER CANCER

The *TP53* Model in Germ Cell Cancer

Germ cell cancer stands out as the most chemosensitive adult solid cancer (Oliver, 1997) apart from choriocarcinoma in females which of course is semi-allogeneic. Figure 4 illustrates how this manifests itself clinically. The fact that close to 100% of patients taking morphine because of pain from metastatic spread are pain free in less than 1 week provides another illustration of the exquisite chemosensitivity.

There is now increasing evidence that the presence of a high frequency of mutation of the *TP53* gene is a factor in the failure to respond to chemotherapy and immunotherapy of the common adult cancers including bladder cancer (Sarkis *et al*, 1995; Lacombe *et al*, 1996). Testis cancer, unlike other cancers, has only rarely been associated with mutation of *TP53* despite being universally associated with overexpression of *TP53* (Peng *et al*, 1993). As the overexpressed *TP53* is in germ cell cancer known to be functional in terms of ability to induce apoptosis if challenged by DNA damaging agents (Huddart *et al*, 1995), this may be an important factor in facilitating the response of these tumours to chemotherapy and radiotherapy. It may even explain the exquisite sensitivity of

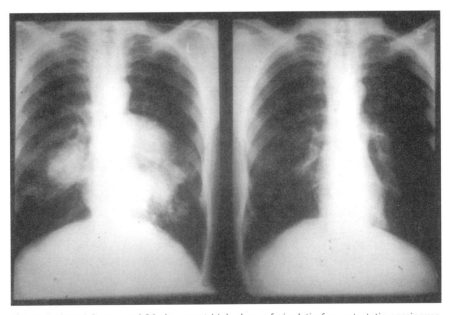

Fig. 4. Patient AC pre- and 21 days post-high dose of cisplatin for metastatic seminoma

normal germ cells to toxic damage that is contributing to declining sperm count in most industrial societies and provide the link with the rising incidence of testis cancer currently observed today (Oliver and Oliver, 1996).

The most important new evidence to help understand this exquisite chemosensitivity and radiosensitivity of these tumours is recently published data showing that normal germ cells switch on *TP53* physiologically during spermatogenesis at the stage of the tetraploid pachytene spermatocyte that precedes meiosis, presumably as a final check of the genome (Schwartz *et al*, 1993). There is increasing evidence (Oliver, 1996) that the stem cell for germ cell cancer may be the same tetraploid pachytene spermatocyte as this cell has the same DNA ploidy values as the premalignant carcinoma in situ (CIS) cell. This is known to have a 50% risk of progression to overt cancer in 5 years. If there was active expression of unmutated functional *TP53* in germ cell cancer at a tetraploid dose, it could play a major part in the unique exquisite chemo-curability of these tumours. There is now increasing evidence that germ cell cancers undergo clonal evolution, and progress from CIS to seminoma and then non-seminoma with loss of DNA content being associated with increasing malignancy (Ooesterhuis *et al*, 1993; Oliver *et al*, 1995). A recent study of snap frozen tissue from 40 germ cell cancers compared to a similar number of bladder and squamous oral cancers demonstrated that *TP53* is easily detected in the majority of germ cell tumours but only in a minority of bladder and squamous oral cancers, while BCL2 and HSP70 expression is generally weak in germ cell cancers but strong and more frequent in bladder and oral squamous cell cancers which are considerably more chemoresistant than germ cell cancers (Table 8).

This study also provided some support for the idea that non-seminomas develop by clonal evolution from CIS cells with combined seminoma malignant teratoma as intermediate between pure seminoma and pure malignant teratoma/non-seminomas (Oliver *et al*, 1995). Though interpretation needs to be guarded because it is based on rather small numbers, *TP53* was more highly expressed in patients with seminoma and combined tumours than pure non-

TABLE 8. Expression of TP53, HSP70 and BCL2 in bladder and testicular germ cell cancer

	No of cases	Positivity	
		Strong (%)	Intermediate/weak (%)
Bladder cancer			
TP53	31	0	7
HSP70	10	60	40
BCL2	10	80	20
Testicular germ cell cancer			
TP53	36	58	30
HSP70	40	12	55
BCL2	40	20	40

seminomas, which are more chemoresistant and express a higher level of BCL2 and HSP70 (Nouri and Oliver, 1997).

Clearly, these observations need more detailed investigation. In particular, given the large amount of data on the role of *TP53* regulation of the mitotic cycle, there is a need for more information on its role in its interaction with other factors regulating the meiotic cell cycle. Taken together with early reports (Fricker, 1996; Roth *et al*, 1996) that intratumoral *TP53* can induce local tumour remissions (Table 6), they give an exciting insight to a possible gene therapy strategy that could be used to increase the sensitivity of metastases from the common solid cancers to chemotherapy. However, what is needed is a mechanism to deliver this construct to the multiple metastatic sites of cancer patients before it can be considered for anything other than an adjuvant role to surgery.

Viral Oncolysis as an Explanation of Renal Cell Cancer Spontaneous Regression

Renal cell cancer has long been known to have one of the highest frequencies of response to immunotherapy but also of spontaneous regression. Because of early worries that chemotherapy might be accelerating renal cell cancer metastases and considerable dispute over the frequency with which spontaneous regression occurred, a Phase 2 study of surveillance prior to treatment was undertaken (Oliver *et al*, 1989b). The response rate was nearly 10 times higher than previous estimates from retrospective studies (Table 9) and this high frequency has been confirmed by more recent studies (Elhilali *et al*, 1997). It was the suggestion that a viral infection had induced tumour lysis in one of our eight patients demonstrating spontaneous regression that led to the renewed interest in this concept. It is more than 30 years since Lindenmann first reported that viral induced lysis of tumour cells produced a vaccine that was capable of inducing bystanding immunity (Lindenmann and Klein, 1967). The patient who demonstrated this phenomenon in our series presented with severe upper abdominal pain and vomiting as well as severely deranged liver function after being disease free for 8 years following nephrectomy for renal vein invasive renal cell cancer. He had been working in Indonesia and returned home feeling extremely ill. Ultrasound revealed liver metastases, which were confirmed on biopsy. Two weeks later his liver function began to improve spontaneously and by 3 months he had normal liver function and computed tomography showed a nearly normal, though not completely normal, liver (Fig. 5). After a remission lasting 12 months his disease recurred and failed to respond to IL2.

A possible interpretation of this patient's history was that he had had slowly growing liver metastases during the 8 years after nephrectomy. It was viral hepatitis that led to them being discovered at an advanced state, but this infection subsequently participated in the lysis of the major part of the established disease. Table 10 summarizes the results from the original paper that led to the

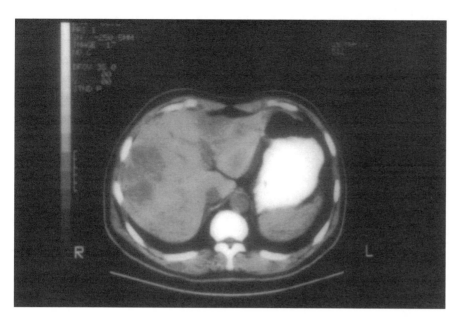

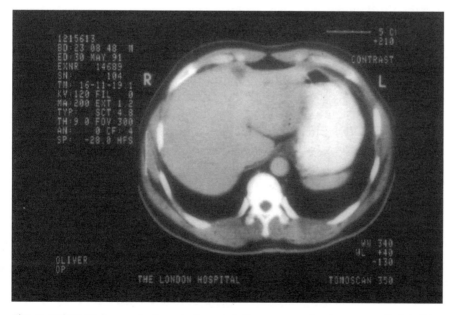

Fig. 5. Patient PS: liver metastases before and after recovery from non-specific "viral" hepatitis acquired in Indonesia

concept of viral oncolysis being proposed by Lindenmann in the early 1960s. Though there were a few clinical trials using such vaccines in an adjuvant setting during the 1970s (Kobayashi, 1979), little work was done using such virus-

TABLE 9. "Unexplained" regression in renal cell cancer*

	No of cases	"Unexplained" regression (%)
Possinger (metastases all)	1247	0.24
Possinger (postnephrectomy)	663	0.6
Bloom	172	1.0
Leahy and Oliver	195	4.1

*For references see Oliver et al (1989b)

es in tumour bearing individuals. Recent progress with low pathogenic recombinant adenovirus (Ko *et al*, 1996) is now making such ideas worth reconsidering.

THE POTENTIAL OF COMBINATION GENE THERAPY

The success of combination chemotherapy has been based on the selection of cancer damaging agents that affect different targets in the cancer cell. Today, progress in genetic engineering means that it is now relatively easy to make constructs of two or three different genes that can be shown to function when expressed together in a cell (Hollingsworth *et al*, 1996). The data reviewed in the previous sections suggest that HLA class I and *TP53* genes have considerable potential when injected into a local tumour mass. It might well be possible to produce a viral construct that incorporated a tetraploid dose of *TP53* as found in germ cell cancer cells and HLA-B7 with a tissue specific promoter that will limit expression in bladder cancer cells. Incorporating such a genetic construct into the viral genome of low pathogenic recombinant adenovirus could provide a way to ensure widespread alterations of a large number of cancer deposits in patients with metastatic disease. It could also be used to lyse tumours in vitro to produce a vaccine for patients at high risk of metastases.

TABLE 10. Viral oncolysis and induction of immunity to Ehrlich ascites tumour (modified from Lindenmann and Klein, 1967)

	No of mice	Survival >40 days (%)
Saline	8	0
Oncolysate*	8	100
Mechanical tumour lysate (MTL)	8	0
Egg-grown virus (EGV)	8	0
MTL + EGV	8	0

*Ehrlich ascites tumour cells 48–72 hours in vitro lysis by WSA strain influenza virus: animals challenged 11 days after vaccination

SUMMARY

In the last decade there has been major progress in understanding the multiple steps involved in cancer cells developing their malignant potential. Study of bladder cancer has provided important information during this period and helped to identify HLA class I and wild type normal *TP53* as potential probes for gene therapy studies.

Given the magnitude of genetic damage that is associated with the clonal development of bladder cancer, and particularly the number of cellular mechanisms that have been highjacked in the development of terminal metastatic disease, it is obviously highly unlikely that a single gene therapy involving HLA class I alone would work in terminal metastatic disease. However, it seems possible that HLA-B7 treatment of patients with bladder cancer who are candidates for salvage cystectomy would benefit such patients. If it were to work, it could provide a whole new approach to managing superficial tumours.

However for patients with extensive metastatic disease, progress could come from investing more effort in uncovering the genetic basis of the chemosensitivity of germ cell tumours and understanding the basis of the normal checkpoints of meiosis and the role of *TP53*. This could provide a completely new approach to gene therapy that might be exploited even in patients with advanced metastatic disease. Such a tetraploidal construct combined with allogeneic HLA class I and incorporated into a low pathogenic lytic viral construct to induce oncolysis with some form of tissue promoter to focus the cell types in which the genes will be activated could provide ideal effective gene therapy.

References

Bicknell D, Kaklamanis L, Hampson R, Bodmer W and Karran P (1996) Selection for beta(2)-microglobulin mutilation in mismatch repair-defective colorectal carcinomas. *Current Biology* **6** 1695–1697

Browning M, Petronzelli F, Bicknell D *et al* (1996) Mechanisms of loss of HLA Class-I expression on colorectal tumor cells. *Tissue Antigens* **47** 364–371

Chan S-Y, Delius H, Halpern A and Bernard HU (1995) Analysis of genomic sequences of 95 papillomavirus types: uniting typing, phylogeny and taxonomy. *Journal of Virology* **69** 3074–3083

Clements VK, Baskar S, Armstrong TD and Ostrand-Rosenberg S (1992) Invariant chain alters the malignant phenotype of MHC class II tumour cells. *Journal of Immunology* **149** 2391

Davies B, Waxman J, Wasan H *et al* et al (1993) Levels of matrix metalloproteases in bladder cancer correlate with tumor grade and invasion. *Cancer Research* **53** 5365–5369

Dickson R and Lippman M (1997) Molecular biology of breast cancer, In: deVita V, Hellman S and Rosenberg S (eds). *Cancer: Principles and Practice of Oncology*, 5th ed, pp 1541–1557, Lippincott-Raven, Philadelphia

Dolin P (1991) An epidemiological review of tobacco use and bladder cancer. *Smoking Related Diseases* **2** 129–143

Elhilali M, Gleave M, Fradet Y *et al* (1997) Placebo-associated remissions in a multicenter randomized double blind trial of interferon gamma 1b (rlFN-y) for the treatment of metastatic renal cell carcinoma (mRCC). *Proceedings of the American Society of Clinical Oncology* **16** [Abstract 1187]

Folkmann J (1990) What is the evidence that tumors are angiogenesis dependent? *Journal of the National Cancer Institute* **82** 4–6

Folkman J and Shing Y (1992) Angiogenesis. *Journal of Biological Chemistry* **267** 10931–10934

Fricker J (1996) Hepatocellular carcinoma and p53 gene therapy. *Molecular Medicine Today* **2** 361

Hollingsworth SJ, Darling D, Gaken J *et al* (1996) The effect of combined expression of interleukin 2 and interleukin 4 on the tumorigenicity and treatment of B16F10 melanoma. *British Journal of Cancer* **74** 6–15

Huddart RA, Titley J, Robertson D, Williams GT, Horwich A and Cooper CS (1995) Programmed cell death in response to chemotherapeutic agents in human germ cell tumour lines. *European Journal of Cancer* **31A** 739–746

Hui K, Grosveld F and Festenstein H (1984) Rejection of transplantable AKR leukaemia cells following MHC DNA-mediated transformation. *Nature* **132** 311

Hui K, Ang P, Huang L and Tay S (1997) Phase 1 study of immunotherapy of cutaneous metastases of human carcinoma using allogeneic MHC-DNA-liposome complexes. *Gene Therapy* **4** 783–790

Hui KM, Sim T, Foo TT and Oei AA (1989) Tumor rejection mediated by transfection with allogeneic class I histocompatibility gene. *Journal of Immunology* **143** 3835–3843

Iles RK, Lee CL, Oliver RTD and Chard T (1990) Composition of intact hormone and free subunits in the human chorionic gonadotrophin-like material found in serum and urine of patients with carcinoma of the bladder. *Clinical Endocrinology* **32** 355–364

Itaya T, Yamagiwa S, Okada F *et al* (1987) Xenogenization of a mouse lung carcinoma (3LL) by transfection with an allogeneic class I major histocompatibility complex gene (H-2Ld). *Cancer Research* **47** 3136–3140

Ito N, Matsuda T, Kakchi Y *et al* (1990) Bladder cancer producing granulocyte colony stimulating factor. *New England Journal of Medicine* **323** 1709–1710

Jaeger TM, Weidner N, Chew K *et al* (1995) Tumor angiogenesis correlates with lymph node metastases in invasive bladder cancer. *Journal of Urology* **154** 69–71

Kaempfer R, Gerez L, Farbstein H *et al* (1996) Prediction of response to treatment in superficial bladder carcinoma through pattern of interleukin-2 gene expression. *Journal of Clinical Oncology* **14** 1778–1786

Kamata S, Kageyama Y, Yonese J and Oshima H (1996) Significant telomere reduction in human superficial transitional cell carcinoma. *British Journal of Urology* **78** 704–708

Ko SC, Gotoh A, Thalmann GN *et al* (1996) Molecular therapy with recombinant p53 adenovirus in an androgen-independent, metastatic human prostate cancer model. *Human Gene Therapy* **7** 1683–1691

Kobayashi H (1979) Viral xenogenization of intact tumor cells. *Advances in Cancer Research* **30** 279–299

Lacombe L, Dalbagni G, Zhang Z *et al* (1996) Overexpression of p53 protein in a high-risk population of patients with superficial bladder cancer before and after Bacillus Calmette-Guerin therapy: correlation to clinical outcome. *Journal of Clinical Oncology* **14** 2646–2652

Lazar V, Diez SG, Laurent A *et al* (1995) Expression of human chorionic gonadotropin beta subunit genes in superficial and invasive bladder carcinomas. *Cancer Research* **55** 3735–3738

Lee SK and Oliver RTD (1978) Autologous leukaemia specific T-cell mediated lymphotoxicity in patients with acute myelogenous leukemia. *Journal of Experimental Medicine* **147** 912–922

Lerner S and Skinner D (1996) Radical cystectomy for bladder cancer, In: Vogelzang N, Scardino P, Shipley W and Coffey D (eds). *Comprehensive Textbook of Genitourinary Oncology*, pp 442–463, Williams & Wilkins, Baltimore

Lindenmann J and Klein PA (1967) Viral oncolysis: increased immunogenicity of host cell antigen associated with influenza virus. *Journal of Experimental Medicine* **126** 93–108

Liotta L (1986) Tumor invasion and metastasis. *Cancer Research* **46** 1

List AF, Miller TP and Grogan TM (1993) Deficient tumor infiltrating T lymphocyte response in malignant lymphoma—relationship to HLA expression and host immunocompetence. *Leukemia* **7** 398–403

Martin ME, Jenkins BJ, Zuk RJ, Oliver RTD and Baithune SI (1989) Human chorionic gonadotrophin expression and histological findings as predictors of response to radiotherapy in carcinoma of the bladder. *Virchows Archiv A, Pathological Anatomy and Histopathology* **414** 273–277

Morin G (1989) The human telomere terminal transferase enzyme is a ribonucleoprotein that synthesizes TTAGGG repeats. *Cell* **59** 521–529

Nabel G, Gordon D, Bishop D *et al* (1996) Transfer of allogeneic major histocompatibility complex and B-2 microglobulin genes with DNA-liposome complexes in human melanoma. *Proceedings of the American Society of Clinical Oncologists.* **15** [Abstract 575]

Nargund V, Yoshida K, Smith J *et al* (1996) Telomerase activity in transitional cell carcinoma; its implications for non-invasive detection of bladder cancer. *British Journal of Urology* **77** 10–11

Neal DE, Marsh C, Bennett MK *et al* (1985) Epidermal-growth-factor receptors in human bladder cancer: comparison of invasive and superficial tumours. *Lancet* **1** 366–368

Nouri AME, Bergbaum A, Lederer E *et al* (1991) Paired tumour infiltrating lymphocyte (TIL) and tumour cell line from bladder cancer: a new approach to study tumour immunology in vitro. *International Journal of Cancer* **27** 608–612

Nouri AME, Hussain RF, Santos AVLD, Gillott DJ and Oliver RTD (1992) Induction of MHC antigens by tumour cell lines in response to interferons. *European Journal of Cancer* **28** 1110–1115

Nouri AME, Hussain FR and Oliver RTD (1994) The frequency of major histocompatibility complex antigen abnormalities in urological tumours and their correction by gene transfection or cytokine stimulation. *Cancer Gene Therapy* **1** 119–123

Nouri AME and Oliver RTD (1997) Tetraploid arrest with overexpressed non-mutated p53 in germ cell cancers: relevance to that chemosensitivity and possible application in non-germ cell cancers. *International Journal of Oncology* **11** 1367–1371

O'Brien T, Cranston D, Fuggle S, Bicknell R and Harris A (1995) Different angiogenic pathways characterize superficial and invasive bladder cancer. *Cancer Research* **55** 510–513

Ohigashi T, Tachibana M, Tazaki H and Nakamura K (1992) Bladder cancer cells express functional receptors for granulocyte-colony stimulating factor. *Journal of Urology* **147** 283–286

Oliver RTD (1976) Histocompatibility matching and renal graft survival. *Proceedings of the Royal Society of Medicine* **69** 531–534

Oliver RTD (1996) Epidemiology of testis cancer, In: Vogelzang N, Shipley W, Scardino P and Coffey D (eds). *Comprehensive Textbook of Genitourinary Oncology,* pp 923–931, Williams & Wilkins, Baltimore, Maryland

Oliver RTD (1997) Future trials in germ cell malignancy (GCM) of the testis. *European Journal of Surgical Oncology* **23** 117–122

Oliver RTD and Lee SK (1978) Histocompatibility antigens and T cell responses to leukaemia antigens, In: Neth RCGR, Hofschneider PH and Mannweiler K (eds). *Modern Trends in Human Leukaemia III*, pp 377–379, Springer-Verlag, Berlin

Oliver RTD and Oliver J (1996) Endocrine hypothesis for declining sperm count and rising testis cancer incidence. *Lancet* **346** 339–340

Oliver RTD, Blandy JP and Hope-Stone HF (1989a) Medical management in bladder cancer, In: *Urological and Genital Cancer*, pp 115–126, Blackwell Scientific Publications, Oxford

Oliver RTD, Nethersall ABW and Bottomley JM (1989b) Unexplained spontaneous regression and alpha-interferon as treatment for metastatic renal carcinoma. *British Journal of Urology* **63** 128–131

Oliver RTD, Nouri AME, Crosby D *et al* (1989c) Biological significance of beta hCG, HLA and other membrane antigen expression on bladder tumours and their relationship to tumour infiltrating lymphocytes (TIL). *Journal of Immunogenetics* **16** 381–390

Oliver RTD, Leahy M and Ong J (1995) Combined seminoma/non-seminoma should be considered as intermediate grade germ cell cancer (GCC). *European Journal of Cancer* **31A** 1392–1394

Ooesterhuis JW, Gillis AJM, van Putten WJL, Jong B and Looijenga LHJ (1993) Interphase cytogenetics of carcinoma in situ of the testis. *European Journal of Urology* **23** 16–22

Peng HQ, Hogg D, Malkin D *et al* (1993) Mutations of the p53 gene do not occur in testis cancer. *Cancer Research* **53** 3574–3578

Pugh R (1973) The pathology of cancer of the bladder: an editorial overview. *Cancer* **32** 1267–1274

Rhyu M (1995) Telomeres, telomerase and immortality. *Journal of the National Cancer Institute* **87** 884–894

Roth JA, Nguyen D, Lawrence DD *et al* (1996) Retrovirus-mediated wild-type p53 gene transfer to tumors of patients with lung cancer. *Nature Medicine* **2** 985–991

Rovere GQD, Oliver RTD, McCance DJ and Castro JE (1988) Development of bladder tumour containing HPV type 11 DNA after renal transplantation. *British Journal of Urology* **62** 36–38

Sarkis A, Bajorin D, Reuter V *et al* (1995) Prognostic value of p53 nuclear overexpression in patients with invasive bladder cancer treated with neoadjuvant M-VAC. *Journal of Clinical Oncology* **13** 1384–1390

Schwartz D, Goldfinger N and Rotter V (1993) Expression of p53 protein in spermatogenesis is confined to the tetraploid pachytene primary spermatocytes. *Oncogene* **8** 1487–1494

Slattery M, Robinson L, Schuman K *et al* (1989) Cigarette smoking and exposure to passive smoke are risk factors for cervical cancer. *Journal of the American Medical Association* **261** 1593–1598

Soloway MS and Masters S (1980) Urothelial susceptibility to tumor cell implantation: influence of cauterization. *Cancer* **46** 1158–1163

Spruck C, Rideout W, Olumi A *et al* (1993) Distinct pattern of p53 mutations in bladder cancer: relationship to tobacco usage. *Cancer Research* **53** 1162–1166

Spruck CH, Ohneseit PF, Gonzalez-Zulueta M *et al* (1994) Two molecular pathways to transitional cell carcinoma of the bladder. *Cancer Research* **54** 784–788

Tomlinson IP and Bodmer WF (1995) The HLA system and the analysis of multifactorial genetic disease. *Trends in Genetics* **11** 493–498

Toshitani K, Braud V, Browning MJ *et al* (1996) Expression of a single-chain HLA class I molecule in a human cell line: presentation of exogenous peptide and processed antigen to cytotoxic T lymphocytes. *Proceedings of the National Academy of Sciences of the USA* **93** 236–240

Vanky F, Wang P, Patarroyo M and Klein E (1990) Expression of the adhesion molecule ICAM-1 and major histocompatibility complex class I antigens on human tumor cells is required for their interaction with autologous lymphocytes in vitro. *Cancer Immunology, Immunotherapy* **31** 19–27

Weldon TE and Soloway MS (1975) Susceptibility of urothelium to neoplastic cellular implantation. *Urology* **5** 824–827

Wilson RW, Chenggis ML and Unger ER (1990) Longitudinal study of human papillomavirus infection of the female urogenital tract by in situ hybridization. *Archives of Pathology and Laboratory Medicine* **114** 155–159

Yoshida K, Sugino T, Tahara H *et al* (1997) Telomerase activity in bladder carcinoma and its implications for noninvasive diagnosis by detection of exfoliated cancer cells in urine. *Cancer* **79** 362–369

Zarling JM, Raich PC, McKeough M and Bach FH (1976) Generation of cytotoxic lymphocytes in vitro against autologous human leukaemia cells. *Nature* **262** 691–693

Zinkernagel RM and Doherty PC (1979) MHC cytotoxic T cells: studies on biological role polymorphic major transplantation antigens determining T cell restriction specificity. *Advanced Immunology* **27** 51

The authors are responsible for the accuracy of the references.

The Role of Surgery in the Multimodality Treatment of Bladder Cancer

MALCOLM J COPTCOAT[1] • R T D OLIVER[2]

[1]Department of Urology, King's College Hospital, London SE5 9RS [2]Department of Medical Oncology, St Bartholomew's Hospital, London EC1A 7BE

Introduction
    The concept of multimodality management of cancer
    History of surgical intervention in bladder cancer
    Histological verification of cancer before multimodality therapy
    Anatomical versus systemic disease hypothesis and failure of radical cancer surgery
    Surgical contribution to evaluation of treatment of superficial disease
Urine cytological washings and pathological staging of bladder cancer
Pathological factors that influence outcome of surgical intervention in bladder cancer
Bladder reconstruction
Neoadjuvant therapy in advanced invasive $T_{3/4}$ and/or node positive tumours
Experimental models of surgery in advanced disease: the justification for early postoperative adjuvant therapy
A surgical perspective on gene therapy
Summary

INTRODUCTION

The debate about the role of surgery in cancer is increasingly in the public's consciousness today. Cancer has only recently become the 20th century version of the "grim reaper" (Hill, 1979). The century began with infectious diseases and particularly tuberculosis in that role. As a result of improved public health, better nutrition and antibiotics they have moved well down the list, at least in developed societies. The commonest killers have become heart disease and cerebrovascular disease, but as preventive measures and successful management of these diseases have produced a generation expecting to live well into their seventies, cancer is now taking a more dominant role. This has in turn stimulated renewed efforts to identify cancers at a very early stage. Why? Because then the "evil that offends thee" can be cut out and the patient supposedly cured. Unfortunately such a simplistic concept is the legacy of heroic surgeons of the past, whose radical and mutilating procedures were seldom

Cancer Surveys Volume 31: *Bladder Cancer*
© 1998 Imperial Cancer Research Fund. 0-87969-529-3/98. $5.00 + .00

129

accompanied by anything other than an even more heroic patient, strangely extremely grateful for their treatment, but still dying of recurrent or metastatic disease. Surgeon and patient alike began to believe that "if only" we had caught the cancer earlier things might have been different.

But even today, despite a wide range of imaging techniques such as computed tomography (CT), magnetic resonance imaging (MRI) and positron emission tomography, we still are not able to pick up most early lesions because visually they differ little from normal surrounding tissues. Cytological assessment of exfoliated cells in urine is a routine investigation, but in practice most urologists set little store by it, because of its low sensitivity. Because of this, the chances of achieving early diagnosis for all cancers is low. Animal tumour models suggest that the spread of malignant cells frequently occurs before a tumour volume has reached a cubic millimetre. Although current management of a locally invasive bladder cancer via a radical cystectomy does seem to cure some patients, and this may reflect an efficient immune system, the majority still die from metastatic disease in the absence of local recurrence. This is presumed to be the result of missed micrometastatic disease at the time of presentation.

Today, few surgeons question whether the scalpel should be the automatic first line approach for all potentially operable cancer, since there is little doubt that more cancer is cured by surgery than by any other modality. Patients cured by surgery alone are predominantly those with slow growing well-differentiated tumours that have not mutated to the metastatic phenotype. The challenge for surgery in the next decade is how to prove the worth of integrating surgery with regional modalities such as radiotherapy and systemic modalities such as chemotherapy and immunotherapy into a multimodality primary management programme. Though this view implies that less surgery will be done for primary diagnostic purposes, it must be remembered that even in tumours with effective systemic treatment modalities, such as testis cancer, surgery has an even more important role in defining when complete response has been achieved and when it is safe to stop debilitating systemic therapy (Oliver *et al*, 1983).

Bladder cancer provides a particularly good illustration of the problems of realising this priority, and this chapter reviews the progress made in this direction.

The Concept of Multimodality Management of Cancer

The management of bladder cancer has traditionally been performed in a uni-modality linear fashion. This has applied to both superficial and invasive cancer. The majority of patients present with painless haematuria and are immediately referred to a surgeon or urologist, certainly in Western Europe and the USA. Delay in investigation of bladder cancer has been well established as being associated with a more advanced disease. Although dipstick haematuria screening is far from routine, when used in high risk situations it is associated with less advanced presentations. Following an intravenous urogram, possibly urine cytology and a cystoscopic biopsy, surgery in either a minimally invasive or radical form was the initial curative procedure. The surgeon then followed the patient until a local recurrence or distant metastasis appeared. At the reappearance of anything other than a superficial recurrence, or when surgical resection was impossible, the patient was referred for radiotherapy. There then followed a course of either palliative radiation therapy or, in some cases, more definitive radiation therapy with curative intent. The radiotherapist then followed the patient long term or until a further recurrence or metastasis necessitated additional treatment. Finally the patient would have been referred to an oncologist for consideration of palliative chemotherapy. In an era in which therapeutic options for cancer care were modest, this unimodality linear approach to treatment was highly functional. However, over the past 20 years changing therapeutic strategies have led to a multimodality therapy for many cancers and have rendered the linear care model obsolete. The impact of such a multidisciplinary approach on survival is best illustrated by the report on ovarian cancer management in Scotland (Junor *et al*, 1994). A retrospective study of 533 cases registered in 1987 was carried out with adjustments for age, stage, pathology, degree of differentiation and presence of ascites. Survival was significantly better regardless of other risk factors with management by a multidisciplinary team.

A variety of factors that are not specifically cancer related help to improve the impact of the multidisciplinary approach and have an important role in the overall therapeutic approach to the cancer patient. Not least of these is the ability of a team with experience and better understanding of prognosis to overcome the patient's fear of death that the word cancer evokes. However, other aspects of the general care of cancer patients are important, such as anaesthetists specializing in pain control and palliative care nurses. These play an important part in both the hospital and community in breaking down the barriers of fear connected with the patient's diagnosis. These professionals are sensitive to the individual and family's psychological needs, as well as those minor adjustments in the home setting, all of which help to improve the quality of the terminal care.

History of Surgical Intervention in Bladder Cancer

The earliest discussion of surgical treatment of tumours (Hill, 1979; Wong and DeCosse, 1990) appears in the ES Papyrus (circa 1600 BC, but it is believed to be based on earlier writings dating back to 3000 BC). The goal of the cancer surgeon has always been to operate electively, without pain and in the belief that early intervention carries with it a higher rate of success. The development of anaesthesia and antisepsis made elective surgical techniques for the treatment of cancer much more acceptable, and rapid developments in cancer surgery began to occur during the second half of the 19th century as tumour specific elective surgery was developed and refined. Before this a surgeon's role in cancer management was to ablate growths using resection or cauterization, limited to tumours of the extremities and other surface structures such as the breast. In those days even simple amputations were accompanied by high rates of mortality secondary to infection, although other factors such as nutrition and poverty were important, as illustrated by the fluctuations in Glasgow's amputation mortality rate, which was shown to correlate inversely with the city's relative prosperity (Hamilton, 1982).

Whereas the early 19th century was a period devoted predominantly to descriptive anatomy and to discoveries in physiology, it was also the period that marked the first report of an industrial cancer, when Percival Pott in 1875 described the occurrence of cancer of the scrotum in chimneysweeps. Ephrain McDowell is also credited with performing the first elective abdominal tumour resection in 1809, when he removed a gigantic ovarian mass weighing 22 pounds. The patient lived another 30 years!

The first reference to surgery of bladder cancer was made by Albarran (1892), who reviewed ten patients undergoing suprapubic operations for bladder tumours. These included ligation or clamping of the pedunculated tumours and excision or piecemeal avulsion of sessile growths. Murphy (1972) reviewed the early history of bladder cancer surgery. Desnos (1896) emphasized the importance of removing a margin of normal mucosa with the tumours. High frequency currents were used by Beer in 1910 for the suprapubic excision and fulguration of bladder tumours, and special ball, plate and loop electrodes were designed for these techniques. While these advances in ablative surgery were being accomplished, the endoscopic assessment and treatment of bladder tumours was developing rapidly. Grunfeld, in 1885, was able to fragment and remove a bladder tumour by means of a transurethral snare. Nitze's operating cystoscope of 1896 was equipped with a similar snare but had the obvious advantage that the surgeon could see and not just feel what he was doing.

The first total cystectomy for bladder cancer was performed in 1887 by Bardenheuer of Cologne. The bladder tumour involved both ureters. His intention was to implant both ureters into the bowel, an operation he had practised on animals, but he was unable to locate one ureter and so left them both draining into the pelvis. The patient died on the fourteenth postoperative day. Pawlick of Prague carried out the first successful cystectomy in 1888 for papillomatosis of the bladder three weeks after he had successfully anastomosed the ureters to the vagina. The patient was well 16 years later (Murphy, 1972).

Histological Verification of Cancer before Multimodality Therapy

Surgical excision remains the simplest diagnostic procedure for most primary tumours. Under these circumstances histopathology classification plays an important part in prognosis based on morphology and tumour markers as well as confirmation that the cancer is confined to the local or regional tissues in the excised specimen. The increasing focus on multimodality therapy in cancer has been made possible partly because of a remarkable advance in imaging technology to improve the execution and outcome of selective biopsy procedures. As well as improved endoscopic instruments for diagnosis of lung, oesophageal, stomach, large bowel and bladder cancers, CT, ultrasonography and MRI are now increasingly used to enhance needle guidance and placement in deep seated tumours. These techniques have improved the accuracy and safety of needle placement and enable either needle aspiration or needle core biopsy to be obtained. The increasing reliability of immunocytochemical and molecular diagnostic techniques has greatly improved the histopathologist's ability to prognosticate on the basis of small tissue samples.

For bladder cancer endoscopic diagnosis is the most frequently used method, since this cancer rarely presents with symptomatic metastatic disease and a less than obvious primary. The advances in endoscopy have allowed extremely accurate visualization of the bladder. In addition the utilization of fibreoptic instruments allows repeated examination under local anaesthesia to monitor response to therapy, which is a considerable advance for developing new therapies. Cold cup biopsies can be taken through either rigid or flexible cystoscopes, and it is common practice to obtain biopsies from the tumour and the tumour base, to determine presence or absence of muscle invasion, as well as from surrounding and distant normal looking epithelium to score for presence and extent of carcinoma-in-situ. A great deal of information can be gained from the visual appearance of a bladder tumour. Papillary lesions are commonly superficial, and for such tumours the surgeon will usually proceed to a complete resection with a specially designed resectoscope.

This surgical procedure, called a transurethral resection of bladder tumours (TURBT) has traditionally been used only for "superficial" disease (T_a, T_1) that does not invade the muscle wall. Until recently it was not considered suitable for the effective treatment of muscle invasive disease because of previously reported poor survival associated with metastases and local recurrence. Hall (1996) was the first to take advantage of modern instruments and challenge this established viewpoint by combining a radical TURBT with systemic chemotherapy. Compared with the use of radical cystectomy, this provided the theoretical advantage of preserving bladder and sexual potency. An additional potential gain from this approach was a shorter operating time, reducing the degree of immune suppression. Gain from this latter concept has been difficult to prove in human studies, though it has been easy to demonstrate in animal models of metastatic disease. Although the series recently reported by Hall failed to show a statistically significant advantage compared with a contemporary series given conventional treatment, his approach was associated with a better quality of life and is increasingly accepted by surgeons. This could become universal if current developments in local approaches to gene therapy can be applied to provide a reliable way to downstage bladder tumour before resection, as is now beginning to emerge from use of local *TP53* gene therapy in lung cancer (Roth *et al*, 1996; Swisher *et al*, 1997).

What is now becoming apparent from a modern understanding of the role of molecular biology and genetics in the clonal development of cancer, and is the raison d'être for this book, is that a particular patient's cancer is rarely a static force. The clonal progression of a patient's disease means that periodical histological reassessment of a patient's cancer, with timely sequential interventions involving surgery, or surgery in combination with endoscopic imaging techniques, may be necessary to get up to date pathological phenotyping to select the appropriate gene for gene therapy. If one metastasis develops by clonal evolution from another and not from a primary, then the information gained from the original operation, which is sometimes the only source of material, could be misleading in selection of appropriate molecular therapy.

Anatomical versus Systemic Disease Hypothesis and Failure of Radical Cancer Surgery

Breast cancer has proved the strongest argument against radical surgery, with superradical and radical mastectomy failing to improve overall cure over lumpectomy (Lacour *et al*, 1983). For the last two decades it has been argued that this is because cancer is a systemic disease and metastasis is present before surgery. With monoclonal antibody and polymerase chain reaction techniques detecting circulating cancer cells in blood and bone marrow of patients with apparently localized cancer such as breast (Johnson *et al*, 1995), prostate (Eschwege *et al*, 1995) and melanoma (Smith *et al*, 1991) the systemic disease hypothesis would seem sound. However, over the past few years a number of factors have begun to question these conclusions and draw attention to local factors induced by surgical intervention that may also be contributing to reducing the gain from radical surgery (Oliver, 1995). The fact that the overall survival is unchanged despite significantly reduced local recurrence rate after radical surgery suggests that occult disease may be accelerated by surgery, eliminating the gain from improved local control. In breast cancer it has been observed that surgery during the oestrogenic phase of the menstrual cycle may accelerate development of metastases, and the more radical the treatment the more marked this effect (Fentiman and Gregory, 1993). This provides an important clue as to how trauma induced tumour cell stimulating growth factors could contribute to undermining the benefits of radical surgery. The demonstration in experimental animals that surgical trauma induces epithelial growth factor release as part of the tissue repair cytokine response (Alexander *et al*, 1988) provides another demonstration of the same principle. This could explain why as long ago as 1910 Peyton Rous observed that tumour cells implanted at sites of surgical trauma demonstrated accelerated growth (Joynes and Rous, 1914) and more recent papers that tumours expressing epidermal growth factor receptor (EGFR) have a poor prognosis after surgery (Qureshi *et al*, this volume). The observation that treatment with anti EGF antibody reduces tumour cell implantation at sites of trauma provides a new direction that might increase the gain from radical surgery in locally advanced cancers. An alternative strategy might be to use tumor necrosis factor alpha (TNFA) since Slooter *et al* (1995) have demonstrated that this treatment blocks the accelerated growth rate of colorectal carcinomas after partial hepatectomy.

The observation that surgery is also associated with a period of postoperative immunosuppression and that the degree of this is proportional to the duration of operation (Oliver *et al*, 1991) demonstrates that there are effects of surgery on tumour growth other than on tissue repair cytokines. It also provides a scientific rationale for the fact that surgical expertise can be so variable that there is a tenfold difference in frequency of local recurrence after such routine surgery as removal of a rectal cancer (Mollen *et al*, 1997) and why there is a similar difference in the operative mortality after radical cystectomy for bladder cancer. At the practical level, these observations also provide a justification for why improved surgical technique from site specialization and setting of standards as to what constitutes adequate referral practice is part of the Calman/Hine reforms of the UK cancer services, with focus on cancer unit/cancer centre splitting of care (Department of Health, 1997).

Surgical Contribution to Evaluation of Treatment of Superficial Disease

There are at least three physical methods by which surgeons can control superficial tumours, ie transurethral diathermy resection, closed cystodiathermy and laser. There are no randomized trials to evaluate the relative merits of these approaches, although it is now more than 20 years since the first suggestion that transurethral diathermy might increase local bladder wall tumour cell implantation (Page *et al*, 1978), which was established by animal studies shortly afterwards (Weldon and Soloway, 1975; Soloway and Masters, 1980). Indirect support for the idea that this risk is real comes from the demonstration that one or three immediate intravesical chemotherapy treatments after TURBT significantly reduce the risk of recurrence at subsequent follow-up (Tolley *et al*, 1996). This evidence and the increased confidence that immunotherapy with BCG leads to a real increase in 10 year survival (Herr *et al*, 1995) should encourage urologists to utilize the considerable ease of access they have to the tumour using flexible cystoscopy and bladder washes to develop experimental approaches to both vaccine and gene therapy treatments (see Nouri *et al*, this volume).

URINE CYTOLOGICAL WASHINGS AND PATHOLOGICAL STAGING OF BLADDER CANCER

There is increasing recognition of the importance of flat carcinoma-in-situ as a precursor of the more life threatening invasive bladder cancer. In the past it has been possible to grow these cells from bladder washings in agar and analyse them with flow cytometry. Today new progress in understanding the cytogenetics of these tumours is opening up the need for greater precision in diagnosis (Knowles, this volume), which could be facilitated if bladder washings provided easy access to cells for typing and prognostication. The development of 24 colour fluorescent in situ hybridization of cytogenetic test to study all 24 chromosomes (Schrock *et al*, 1996) is offering a particularly exciting approach that could be performed using cytological washings rather than diathermy traumatized pieces of tumour because of the need to get mitotic figures.

Loss of part or all of chromosome 9 is the most common molecular genetic event, occurring in 319 (55%) of 580 bladder tumours reported (Spruck *et al*, 1994). This high frequency and the fact that it occurs in both low grade low stage tumours and high grade high stage tumours strongly suggest that loss of one or more suppressor genes on chromosome 9 is an early event. Chromosome 17p is deleted in over 40% of cases, reflecting probable inactivation of the *TP53* suppressor gene. Loss of chromosome 13q occurs in 20% of cases, probably reflecting inactivation of the retinoblastoma suppressor gene. More important than the relatively high frequencies of chromosome 9 and *TP53* alterations in bladder cancer are their differing frequencies in the two distinct morphological types of non-invasive and superficial bladder cancer, ie papillary transitional cell carcinoma (TCC) and flat dysplastic carcinoma-in-situ lesions. The sequence of early molecular alterations before development of invasive disease is different in these two groups. In non-invasive low grade papillary TCC and in low grade T_1 cancers, that is those that have penetrated the lamina propria, allelic losses of chromosome 9 are common, whereas *TP53* mutations are rare. Progression of superficial papillary TCC and low grade T_1 cancers to either a higher grade or a muscle invasive stage is a very uncommon event and is usually accompanied by a mutation in *TP53*. By contrast *TP53* mutations have been found in over two thirds of carcinoma-in-situ lesions, a form of the disease that commonly progresses to invasive cancer.

These differences support a proposed two pathway model for the pathogenesis and progression of bladder cancer. Inactivation of the *TP53* suppressor gene early in tumorigenesis appears to lead to a high degree of genetic instability, the rapid and frequent accumulation of additional genetic alterations, especially loss of chromosome 9, and the high propensity of carcinoma-in-situ lesions to progress to invasive cancer compared with other superficial tumours. By contrast the chromosome 9 defect observed primarily in superficial papillary and minimally invasive low grade tumours may be less destabilizing as an early event than loss of *TP53* suppressor function, since fewer than 20% of these tumours ultimately progress to muscle invasive disease. In the final pathway allelic losses of chromosome 9 can be found in approximately 60% of muscle invasive bladder cancers (T_2, T_3 and T_4), and *TP53* mutations can be documented in 50%.

Furthermore, loss of *TP53* suppressor function conveys a highly aggressive behaviour to carcinoma-in-situ lesions, as reflected in the significantly poorer survival of patients with organ confined bladder cancers bearing this molecular marker than those without *TP53* mutations. Esrig (1994) has demonstrated that the mutational status of *TP53* was the most important prognostic factor, outweighing T stage and grade, associated with disease free survival in a group of 243 patients with surgically staged organ confined bladder cancer (Esrig *et al*, 1994). The disease free survival of patients with wild type compared to mutated *TP53* in this group was 93% vs 78% for pathological stage PT_1, 79% vs 30% for PT_2, 64% vs 22% for PT_{3A}, 52% vs 27% for PT_{3B} and 57% vs 0% for PT_4. Thus as in the well studied models of colorectal tumorigenesis the timing and ordering of genetic defects in bladder cancer play an extremely important part in determining biological behaviour as well as pathogenesis.

PATHOLOGICAL FACTORS THAT INFLUENCE OUTCOME OF SURGICAL INTERVENTION IN BLADDER CANCER

Despite the multiplicity of new molecular markers of prognosis in bladder cancer, it is still the presence of lymph node metastases and the demonstration of invasion of bladder wall muscle that are the two most frequent pathological risk factors routinely used to determine prognosis and the need for additional treatment (Droller and Gosodarowicz, 1996). Because of the deep seated position of the bladder, it is only after major surgical intervention that it is possible to identify these variables. If surgeons are to gain significant benefit from multimodality therapy there is a need to validate prognostic factors that determine prognosis before surgical intervention. As both node status and muscle invasion correlate with tumour grade, molecular markers of high grade tumour such as *TP53* mutation, HLA antigen loss, EFGR and B human chorionic gonadotropin expression are alternative surrogates that could be used. Prospective validation of the use of these markers as positive predictors of prognosis to determine the need for neoadjuvant therapy before surgico-pathological staging will be an important priority for future trials.

Node status stands out as the most significant predictor of poor outcome in bladder cancer, as it does in almost all surgically treatable cancers such as breast, colon, lung, stomach, head and neck and melanoma. Despite this predictive value, the failure of randomized trials in breast cancer (Stewart *et al*, 1989) and melanoma (Veronesi, 1987) to demonstrate any value from routine surgical removal of draining nodes is one of the paradoxes of the debate over radical vs minimal surgery in cancer. There is little doubt that some patients with positive nodes are cured following complete removal of affected nodes. This benefit is least disputed in patients with low stage non-seminomatous germ cell cancers of the testis (clinical stages I and II) who were found to have positive para-aortic nodes at the time of primary lymphadenectomy. Even without adjuvant chemotherapy, 50% of such patients remain disease free (Williams *et al*, 1987). However, because chemotherapy is now so effective, short course neoadjuvant treatment and salvage surgery in the 2% who relapse produces more than 98% cure.

The value of surgical removal of involved nodes in bladder cancer is less clearly quantified. There is some clinical evidence, as yet uncontrolled, to suggest in contrast to the results from breast and melanoma, that some patients with invasive bladder cancer and micrometastatic disease in pelvic lymph nodes only can be cured by a cystectomy and complete pelvic lymphadenectomy. Approximately 30% of patients with high grade (G_2 and G_3) bladder cancers have lymph node metastases, and in one study half of these survived 5 years after lymphadenectomy (Lerner et al, 1993). As yet the benefit of this approach has not been quantified in randomized trials. However, compared to historical controls, introduction of this procedure in one centre increased the 5 year survival after surgery alone for high grade T_2 and T_3 bladder cancers from 10% to 40%, though improvements in staging techniques, reduction in anaesthesia and other morbidities have undoubtedly played some part in these improved results.

In addition to the apparent survival advantage for a subgroup of patients with regional lymph node metastasis in undergoing a therapeutic lymphadenectomy, there is evidence from the study of metastases and primary tumour together that in some cases there are additional chromosome aberrations in affected pelvic lymph nodes when compared with the primary tumour. This provides a possible explanation for the varied subsequent aggressiveness of some tumours that present with positive regional nodes. Support for this comes from the observation that cellular composition of different metastases in the same host is heterogeneous, both within a single metastasis (intralesional heterogeneity) and among different metastases (interlesional heterogeneity). This heterogeneity reflects two major processes: the selective nature of the metastatic process and the rapid evolution and phenotypic diversification of clonal tumour cell populations during progressive tumour growth (which itself results from the inherent genetic and phenotypic instability of many clonal populations of tumour cells) (Fidler, 1995).

Despite these observations the need for accurate staging of bladder cancer with respect to nodal status remains controversial. There is little doubt that even today modern imaging techniques are inadequate to define micrometastatic disease in normally sized nodes. There is increasing evidence that day case endoscopic extraperitoneal node dissection can overcome this problem (Mazeman et al, 1992). However, in most centres the information gained has not altered the management of the patient, who will still probably undergo either radical surgery or radical radiotherapy, but perhaps with less optimistic results in mind.

The new data on the benefits of systemic interferon therapy in node positive melanoma (Kirkwood et al, 1996) may possibly change this attitude, if such therapy were to prove beneficial in all solid cancer with node positive disease. Today new techniques using radioactive monoclonal antibody scanning to localize sentinel lymph node metastatic sites in breast (Shriver *et al*, 1997), melanoma (Ross, 1996) and prostate cancer (Chengazi *et al*, 1997) are simplifying diagnosis of node positive patients. There could be a case for developing such an immune endoscopic staging procedure for bladder cancer. As well as being particularly useful to improve the selection of patients for bladder reconstruction surgery, it could improve early diagnosis of node positive cases for study of immunotherapy.

BLADDER RECONSTRUCTION

In the past, radical cystectomy was an operation with high mortality and high morbidity, including guaranteed loss of potency and resulting in a relatively unsightly external spout which had to be contained within a bag. As most patients with invasive cancer were over the age of 65 at the time of diagnosis, few surgeons in the UK felt that routine use of cystectomy was justified, since early trials demonstrated no gain from early surgery in such patients and only borderline benefit in those under 65. The greatest benefit came from the use of cystectomy as salvage procedure after failed radiation (Bloom *et al*, 1982).

The last 20 years have seen remarkable progress in developing techniques of bladder reconstruction (Taylor and Grune, 1996). These techniques either developed a continent stoma in the abdominal wall, which was emptied by catheter, an augmented (to improve compliance) rectal bladder or created a new bladder from a loop of bowel stitched to the external urinary sphincter after the bladder and prostate were removed (Fig. 1). With the development of techniques for conserving the pelvic parasympathetic plexus involved in erection, potency can now also be preserved more frequently.

Because radiation damage to the tissues made the delicate surgery less successful and because local recurrence was highest in node and advanced muscle invasive disease, it soon became apparent that bladder reconstruction surgery was only justifiable for patients with early cancer such as carcinoma-in-situ, multiple recurrent superficial tumours or early invasive disease.

With easier screening for haematuria possible because of instant urine screening tests and simpler approaches to diagnosis with flexible cystoscopy, bladder cancers are today being diagnosed earlier and there are more opportunities for performing bladder reconstruction. Proving that such increased intervention improves survival is extremely difficult. Even in the most expert hands these procedures are not totally complication free, and every surgeon has a learning curve. In addition, there are several variations on a theme, with little consensus on a standard reconstruction technique, to say nothing about precise agreement at which stage the procedure is best performed. Nevertheless orthotopic bladder reconstruction (new bladder made from small or large bowel and joined to the urethra) can now be achieved in both sexes, because the smooth

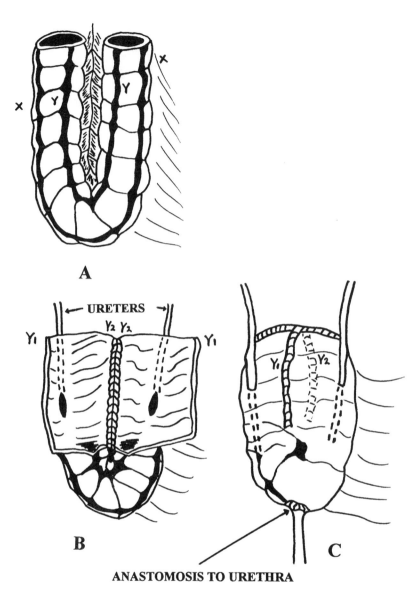

A

← URETERS →

B

C

ANASTOMOSIS TO URETHRA

Fig. 1. Urinary diversion to a new bladder. A, a portion of sigmoid and descending colon measuring 35 cm is isolated and folded in the shape of a U. B, the curve of the U is oriented to the pelvis. The medial taenia of the U is incised down to a point a few centimeters cephalad to the site of the urethral anastomosis. The medial limbs of the U are sutured together, and a tunnelled ureteral implantation is performed (Y2-Y2). C, a button of tissue is removed from the most inferior portion of the pouch, and urethral anastomosis is performed. The pouch is closed by rotating each side of the pouch medially and suturing Y1 to Y2

muscle of the bowel will simulate the behaviour of normal bladder muscle with respect to sensation of filling and usually voiding. Although nearly 25% of patients require revision surgery and 15% may need to self catheterize because of incomplete emptying, the improved quality of life is marked compared to an incontinent stoma.

To devise an acceptable randomized trial to establish the value of early use of such reconstructive surgery would probably be even more difficult than the recent Medical Research Council radical prostatectomy trial for prostate cancer, which failed to recruit. However, the increasingly good results now being achieved by this reconstructive surgery in the hands of experienced surgeons make a strong case for use of such surgery and would be made even stronger by a positive randomized trial. Given the resources consumed by repeated cystoscopy for the high risk patient with persistently recurrent tumour over 10 or more years, health economists could well justify a randomized trial of immediate versus deferred radical surgery in superficial cancer patients whose histology showed high risk features such as *TP53* mutation, loss of blood group antigen or positive EGFR.

NEOADJUVANT THERAPY IN ADVANCED INVASIVE T$_{3/4}$ AND/OR NODE POSITIVE TUMOURS

In all studies in this subgroup of patients the single most significant predictor of survival is treatment induced complete remission (Blandy *et al*, 1980). This occurs in about 30–40% of patients treated with radiation and about 20–30% treated with chemotherapy (Zietman *et al*, 1993). Because of the large number of node positive patients in the subgroup failing radiation or chemotherapy, the potential benefit from radical surgery in these cases is more than offset by the number in whom surgery is abandoned because of inoperability.

There are two aspects of surgery that require examination in this subgroup of patients, the first relates to use of transurethral resection of bladder tumour to minimize tumour bulk. Today this is routinely used before induction therapy whether chemotherapy, radiation or synchronous chemo/radiation therapy (Boshoff *et al*, 1995; Coppin *et al*, 1996). Even with synchronous combination chemotherapy and radiation, more than a third of tumours are resistant to treatment, but if the tumour is resected first it takes much longer to know whether it is resistant. Because of the potential advantages of learning early whether patients have chemo or radiosensitive tumours there could be a case for using such treatment before TURBT. With increasing recognition of the potential risks associated with surgically induced tissue repair cytokine release (Alexander *et al*, 1988) there might even be additional therapeutic advantage in such treatment before TURBT. Treatment induced reduction of tumour bulk would then make endoscopic removal of the whole tumour technically easier and give more information about treatment response from histology. An immediate vs deferred TURBT trial in such patients could provide useful information on the value of histological complete response and accelerate progress in selecting active treatment, as it already has done so clearly in osteogenic sarcoma (Rosen *et al*, 1982).

The second surgical question is whether immediate radical surgery after clinical complete response improves survival. Many reviews have demonstrated a

20–30% understaging and viable cancer at cystectomy in clinical complete responders, and the transitional epithelium of the bladder remains at risk of a second invasive tumour for the rest of the patient's life. There is a need for a trial designed to examine surgery and immediate bladder reconstruction in complete responders versus salvage cystectomy trials. Such a trial could be run in parallel with the similar trial proposed for poor risk superficial tumours.

Given the resources involved in setting up such neoadjuvant trials, preliminary evaluation of such approaches in experimental models looking particularly at healing of tissues after bladder reconstruction in animals treated by induction of chemotherapy/radiotherapy schedules would help to resolve some of the uncertainty about the risks of operative complications after chemo/radiotherapy.

EXPERIMENTAL MODELS OF SURGERY IN ADVANCED DISEASE: THE JUSTIFICATION FOR EARLY POSTOPERATIVE ADJUVANT THERAPY

Laboratory models of adjuvant therapy have been extremely useful for investigating some of the prevalent hypotheses regarding the clinical treatment of micrometastatic disease and the conclusions are equally applicable in bladder cancer. One important observation is that dose intensity is as critical if not more so when used in adjuvant treatment as when such chemotherapy is used in the treatment of advanced metastatic disease alone. Low dose therapy has little value in most cases. There have been several attempts to define mathematically the relationship between drug dose and tumour cell kill. One of the earliest was that of Norton and Simon (1986) who have put forward a model to describe the pattern of growth in solid tumours demonstrating Gompertzian kinetics. Gompertzian growth accounts for variable rates of mitosis in a mass with an ischaemic inner portion of cell dying faster than the tumour can grow and fits in with clinical observations that large masses grow more slowly. The implications of the Norton/Simon model for clinical practice are the following:

The extent of therapy sufficient to cause tumour regression may not be sufficient to eradicate the tumour completely. This is clearly demonstrated by the relapse rate and survival of patients who have achieved a complete response (CR) with methotrexate, vinblastine, adriamycin and cisplatinin (M-VAC).

Treatments that cause regression of large tumours may not necessarily be sufficient to cure small tumours treated in adjuvant protocols, and in these cases chemotherapy dose intensity may be extremely important. Low dose maintenance programmes usually have not been effective clinically for the management of solid tumours, although in breast and bowel cancer there is some evidence that certain cytotoxic agents that are only modestly active in advanced tissue disease might be effective in an adjuvant application (Bonadonna, 1992; IMPACT, 1995). However, even in breast cancer more recent data suggest that there is even more survival advantage from use of ultrahigh dose with stem cells as adjuvant (Peters *et al*, 1993) than when it is used for advanced disease (Bezwoda *et al*, 1995).

A second important conclusion of the laboratory studies is that the timing of therapy appears to be critical. Although adjuvant treatment has traditionally followed surgery, it is important to appreciate that the process of surgical debulking can alter the growth kinetics of metastases. The doubling time of secondary tumour deposits in experimental animals can be altered adversely and survival time can decrease. Clinical surgical debulking in testis cancer has been observed to increase doubling time of metastases (Javadpour *et al*, 1982; Lange *et al*, 1980). Consequently if postoperative adjuvant therapy is chosen the interval between surgery and the start of therapy appears critical. This has been well demonstrated in animal models using the Lillims tumour. That delays of even a few days can alter the ultimate treatment outcome is suggested from the study using single agent cyclophosphamide as adjuvant treatment for breast cancer (Nissen-Meyer *et al*, 1978). These observations suggest that if postoperative therapy is chosen it must be initiated immediately after surgery. Unfortunately this approach is difficult for many surgeons and patients because of postoperative problems. Support for the idea of early initiation of adjuvant therapy has now come from mathematical models developed to study the development of new tumour cell phenotypes (particularly concerning drug resistance) on the basis of inherent rate of spontaneous mutations. These analyses suggest that drug resistance in subpopulations of the tumour occurs early in the progression of the disease. Zonal differences in primary tumours are not restricted to morphology but include biological characteristics such as growth rates, sensitivity/resistance to cytotoxic drugs and antigenicity. In other words, a clone of resistant cells, however small may exist at a very early clinical stage (Fidler and Hart, 1981).

A SURGICAL PERSPECTIVE ON GENE THERAPY

The past decade has seen a rapid explosion in ideas from laboratory animal and in vitro studies of gene therapy that have potential for application in treatment of cancer. The most extensively studied are:

- Enhancement of tumour immunogenicity (eg with foreign antigens, cytokines)
- Genetic alteration of immune cells to increase function (eg cytokines, co-stimulatory molecules)
- Insertion of a "sensitivity" or "suicide" gene into the tumour (eg herpes simplex/thymidine kinase, cytosine deaminase)
- Blocking of oncogene expression (eg antisense *KRAS*, intracellular antibodies)
- Insertion of a tumour suppressor gene (eg wild type *TP53*)

- Protection of tissues from the systemic toxicities of chemotherapy (eg multiple drug resistance type 1 gene)
- Induction of normal tissues to produce antitumour substances (eg interleukin 2, interferon)
- Production of recombinant vaccines for the prevention and treatment of malignancy (eg BCG expressing tumour antigens)
- Local radioprotection of normal bystander tissues with antioxidant overexpression (eg glutathione synthetase or transferase)

The potential of two of these—enhancement of tumour immunogenicity and insertion of a tumour suppressor gene—has been explored by Nouri *et al* (this volume). The vaccine approach in experimental animals with minimal residual disease has been most widely explored. The long history of poor results of postsurgical adjuvant immunotherapy vaccine studies in the past 20 years and, more significantly, the long duration of follow-up needed to prove whether such approaches work casts doubt on the value of such studies at present. Given the multiplicity of approaches and the multiplicity of damaged genes that are now being identified from modern studies of the genetic basis of cancer, it may seem naive to believe that selecting only one gene for manipulation would demonstrate therapeutic benefit. However, given the easy access to the bladder that modern flexible endoscopy offers the urologist and the increasing evidence that there are ways to introduce genes by direct tumour inoculation using viral vectors or liposomes (DNA wrapped in lipid), it is clear that both superficial and invasive bladder cancer are ideal for doing measurable disease studies with gene therapy probes used in a neoadjuvant fashion before local tumour resection to get histological verification of effect. The urologist will have a critically important role in the development of such studies.

SUMMARY

There has been little change in bladder cancer survival for more than 40 years, although earlier diagnosis is now detecting more cases at an early, potentially curable stage. Radical cystectomy remains the most effective single treatment, although in the past the morbidity and mortality of treatment and the age of patients made it less favoured as primary treatment. Progress in continent bladder reconstruction is changing attitudes. However, because tissue damage from preoperative radiation, particularly when combined with chemotherapy, makes such operations less safe in patients with advanced disease, reconstruction is primarily of value in high risk superficial and early invasive cancers, though there remains a need for randomized trials or immediate vs deferred use of these operations to establish when they give most benefit.

With new knowledge about the role of trauma released tissue repair cytokines and immunosuppressive effect of prolonged anaesthesia on increasing tumour recurrence after surgery, new approaches such as treatment with TNFA, anti-EGF antibody or neoadjuvant chemo/immunotherapy before

TURBT to improve on the benefits of surgery need to be explored in randomized trials in both advanced invasive and early superficial disease.

With progress in vaccine and gene therapy on the horizon, the central role of the urologist in both harvesting tumours for molecular diagnosis and monitoring response of local disease to treatment is undisputed. The relative under-usage and value of bladder washings cytology to provide cells for such studies is also highlighted.

References

Albarran J (1892) *Les Tumeurs de la Vessie*, G Steinheil, Paris

Alexander P, Murphy P and Skipper D (1988) Preferential growth of blood borne cancer cells at site of trauma: a growth promoting role of macrophages. *Advances in Experimental Medicine and Biology*

Alexander P, Murphy P and Skipper D (1988) Preferential growth of blood borne cancer cells at site of trauma: a growth promoting role of macrophages. *Advances in Experimental Medicine and Biology* **233** 245–251

Bezwoda WR, Seymour L and Dansey RD (1995) High-dose chemotherapy with hematopoietic rescue as primary treatment for metastatic breast cancer: a randomized trial. *Journal of Clinical Oncology* **13** 2483–2489

Blandy JP, England HR, Evans SJW *et al* (1980) T$_3$ bladder cancer: the case for salvage cystectomy. *British Journal of Urology* **52** 506–510

Bloom HJ, Hendry WF, Wallace DM and Skeet RG (1982) Treatment of T$_3$ bladder cancer: controlled trial of pre-operative radiotherapy and radical cystectomy versus radical radiotherapy. *British Journal of Urology* **54** 136–151

Bonadonna G (1992) Evolving concepts in the systemic adjuvant treatment of breast cancer. *Cancer Research* **52** 2127–2137

Boshoff C, Gallagher CJ, Oliver RTD *et al* (1995) A pilot study of combination chemotherapy with concurrent radiotherapy in patients with locally advanced bladder cancer. *Proceedings of the American Society of Clinical Oncology* **14** 249 [Abstract 670]

Chengazi VU, Feneley MR, Ellison D *et al* (1997) Imaging prostate cancer with technetium-99m-7E11-C5 3 (CYT-351). *Journal of Nuclear Medicine* **38** 675–682

Coppin C, Gospodarowicz MK, James K *et al* (1996) Improved local control of invasive bladder cancer by concurrent cisplatin and preoperative or definitive radiation. *Journal of Clinical Oncology* **14** 2901–2907

Department of Health (1997) *Policy Framework for Cancer Services*, Department of Health, London

Droller MJ and Gosodarowicz MK (1996) Staging of bladder cancer, In: Vogelzang N, Scardino P, Shipley W and Coffey D (eds). *Comprehensive Textbook of Genitourinary Oncology*, pp 359–370, Williams & Wilkins, Baltimore

Eschwege P, Dumas F, Blanchet P *et al* (1995) Haematogenous dissemination of prostatic epithelial cells during radical prostatectomy. *Lancet* **346** 1528–1529

Esrig D, Elmajian D, Groshen S *et al* (1994) Accumulation of nuclear p53 and tumor progression in bladder cancer. *New England Journal of Medicine* **331** 1259–1264

Fentiman IS and Gregory WM (1993) The hormonal milieu and prognosis in operable breast cancer. *Cancer Surveys* **18** 149–163

Fidler IJ (1995) Invasion and metastasis, In: Abeloff P (ed). *Invasion and Metastasis in Clinical Oncology*, pp 55–76, Churchill Livingstone, London

Fidler IJ and Hart IR (1981) Biological and experimental consequences of the zonal composition of solid tumors. *Cancer Research* **41** 3266–3267

Hall RR (1996) The role of transurethral surgery alone and with combined modality therapy, In: Vogelzang N, Scardino P, Shipley W and Coffey D (eds). *Comprehensive Textbook of Genitourinary Oncology*, pp 509–522, Williams & Wilkins, Baltimore

Hamilton DNH (1982) The nineteenth century surgical revolution: antisepsis or better nutrition. *Bulletin of Historial Medicine* **56** 30–40

Herr HW, Schwalb DM, Zhang ZF *et al* (1995) Intravesical bacillus Calmette-Guerin therapy prevents tumor progression and death from superficial bladder cancer: ten-year follow-up of a prospective randomized trial. *Journal of Clinical Oncology* **13** 1404–1408

Hill GJD (1979) Historic milestones in cancer surgery. *Seminars in Oncology* **6** 409–427

IMPACT (1995) International multicentre pooled analysis of colon cancer trials: efficacy of adjuvant fluorouracil and folinic acid in colon cancer. *Lancet* **345** 935–944

Javadpour N, Ozols RF, Anderson T *et al* (1982) A randomized trial of cytoreductive surgery followed by chemotherapy versus chemotherapy alone in bulky stage testicular cancer with poor prognostic features. *Cancer* **50** 2004–2010

Johnson P, Burchill S and Selby P (1995) The molecular detection of circulating tumour cells. *British Journal of Cancer* **72** 268–276

Joynes F and Peyton R (1914) On the cause of localisation of secondary tumour at points of injury. *Journal of Experimental Medicine* **20** 404–412

Junor EJ, Hole DJ and Gillis CR (1994) Management of ovarian cancer: referral to a multidisciplinary team matters. *British Journal of Cancer* **70** 363–370

Kirkwood JM, Strawderman MH, Ernstoff MS *et al* (1996) Interferon alfa-2b adjuvant therapy of high-risk resected cutaneous melanoma: the Eastern Cooperative Oncology Group trial EST 1684. *Journal of Clinical Oncology* **14** 7–17

Lacour J, Le M, Caceres E *et al* (1983) Radical mastectomy versus radical mastectomy plus internal mammary dissection. Ten year results of an international cooperative trial in breast cancer. *Cancer* **51** 1941–1943

Lange PH, Hekmat K, Bosl G, Kennedy BJ and Fraley EE (1980) Accelerated growth of testicular cancer after cytoreductive surgery. *Cancer* **45** 1498–1506

Lerner SP, Skinner DG, Lieskovsky G *et al* (1993) The rationale for en bloc pelvic lymph node dissection for bladder cancer patients with nodal metastases: long-term results. *Journal of Urology* **149** 758–764; discussion 764–765

Mazeman E, Wurtz A, Gilliot P and Biserte J (1992) Extraperitoneal pelvioscopy in lymph node staging of bladder and prostatic cancer. *Journal of Urology* **147** 366–370

Mollen RM, Damhuis RA and Coebergh JW (1997) Local recurrence and survival in patients with rectal cancer, diagnosed 1981–1986: a community hospital-based study in the south-east Netherlands. *European Journal of Surgical Oncology* **23** 20–23

Murphy LJT (1972) *The History of Urology*, CC Thomas, Springfield, Illinois

Nissen-Meyer R, Kjellgren K, Malmio K *et al* (1978) Surgical adjuvant chemotherapy results with one short course with cyclophosphamide after mastectomy for breast cancer. *Cancer* **41** 2088–2098

Norton L and Simon R (1986) The Norton-Simon hypothesis revisited. *Cancer Treatment Report* **70** 163–169

Oliver RTD (1995) Does surgery disseminate or accelerate cancer? *Lancet* **346** 1506–1507

Oliver RTD, Blandy JP, Hendry WF *et al* (1983) Evaluation of radiotherapy and/or surgico-pathological staging after chemotherapy in the management of metastatic germ cell tumours. *British Journal of Urology* **55** 764–768

Oliver RTD, Riddle P and Blandy JP (1991) Operative factors and tumour membrane antigen changes in escape from immune surveillance of bladder cancer. *Progress in Clinical and Biological Research* **370** 161–168

Page BH, Levison VB and Curwen MP (1978) The site of recurrence of non-infiltrating bladder tumours. *British Journal of Urology* **50** 237–242

Peters WP, Ross M, Vredenburgh JJ *et al* (1993) High-dose chemotherapy and autologous bone marrow support as consolidation after standard-dose adjuvant therapy for high-risk primary breast cancer. *Journal of Clinical Oncology* **11** 1132–1143

Rosen G, Caparros B, Huvos AG *et al* (1982) Preoperative chemotherapy for osteogenic sarcoma: selection of postoperative adjuvant chemotherapy based on the response of the primary tumor to preoperative chemotherapy. *Cancer* **49** 1221–1230

Ross MI (1996) Surgical management of stage I and II melanoma patients: approach to the regional lymph node basin. *Seminars in Surgical Oncology* **12** 394–401

Roth JA, Nguyen D, Lawrence DD *et al* (1996) Retrovirus-mediated wild-type p53 gene transfer to tumours of patients with lung cancer. *Nature Medicine* **2** 985–991

Schrock E, duManoir S, Veldman T *et al* (1996) Multicolor spectral karyotyping of human chromosomes. *Science* **273** 494–497

Shriver C, Balingit AG, Caravalho J *et al* (1997) Unfiltered Tc-99m sulfur colloid lymphoscintigraphy and gamma-probe in detection of sentinel node in breast cancer patients. *Journal of Nuclear Medicine,* (Supplement on Proceedings of the 4th Annual Meetingof Int. Soc. Nuclear Medicine) [Abstract 119]

Slooter GD, Marquet RL, Jeekel J and Ijzermans JN (1995) Tumour growth stimulation after partial hepatectomy can be reduced by treatment with tumour necrosis factor alpha. *British Journal of Surgery* **82** 129–132

Smith B, Selby P, Southgate J *et al* (1991) Detection of melanoma cells in peripheral blood by means of reverse transcriptase and polymerase chain reaction. *Lancet* **338** 1227–1229

Soloway MS and Masters S (1980) Urothelial susceptibility to tumor cell implantation: influence of cauterization. *Cancer* **46** 1158–1163

Spruck CH, Ohneseit PF, Gonzalez-Zulueta M *et al* (1994) Two molecular pathways to transitional cell carcinoma of the bladder. *Cancer Research* **54** 784–788

Stewart HJ, Prescott RJ and Forrest PA (1989) Conservation therapy of breast cancer. *Lancet* **ii** 168–169

Swisher SG, Roth JA, Lawrence DD *et al* (1997) Adenoviral-mediated p53 gene transfer in patients with advanced non-small cell lung cancer (NSCLC). *Proceedings of the American Society of Clinical Oncology,* **16** [Abstract 1565]

Taylor RJ and Grune MT (1996) Urinary diversions and reconstruction: introduction and standards, In: Vogelzang N, Scardino P, Shipley W and Coffey D (eds). *Comprehensive Textbook of Genitourinary Oncology,* pp 472–479, Williams & Wilkins, Baltimore

Tolley DA, Parmar MKB, Grigor KM, Lallemand G and MRC Superficial Bladder Cancer Working Party (1996) The effect of intravesical mitomycin C on recurrence of newly diagnosed superficial bladder cancer: a further report with 7 years of follow up. *Journal of Urology* **155** 1233–1238

Veronesi U (1987) Delayed node dissection in stage one malignant melanoma: justification and advantages. *Cancer Investigations* **5** 47–53

Weldon TE and Soloway MS (1975) Susceptibility of urothelium to neoplastic cellular implantation. *Urology* **5** 824–827

Williams SD, Stablein DM, Einhorn LH *et al* (1987) Immediate adjuvant chemotherapy versus observation with treatment at relapse in pathological stage. II, testicular cancer. *New England Journal of Medicine* **317** 1433

Wong RJ and DeCosse JJ (1990) Cytoreductive surgery. *Surgery Gynecology and Obstetrics* **170** 276–281

Zietman AL, Shipley WU and Kaufman DS (1993) The combination of cisplatin based chemotherapy and radiation in the treatment of muscle-invading transitional cell cancer of the bladder. *International Journal of Radiation Oncology Biology Physics* **27** 161–170

The authors are responsible for the accuracy of the references.

Radiotherapy and Chemotherapy for Invasive Bladder Cancer

MILAND JAVLE • DEREK RAGHAVAN*

Departments of Solid Tumor Oncology and Investigational Therapeutics, Roswell Park Cancer Institute, Buffalo; and State University of New York, Buffalo, NY

Introduction
Radiotherapy
Concurrent chemoradiation
Systemic chemotherapy for invasive bladder cancer
    Neoadjuvant chemotherapy
    Adjuvant chemotherapy
Future prospects
Summary

INTRODUCTION

Invasive bladder cancer represents only about 20% of cases of newly diagnosed bladder cancer and consists predominantly of transitional cell carcinoma, sometimes intermingled with elements of squamous carcinoma and/or adenocarcinoma. With the increasing emphasis on bladder conservation for patients with superficial bladder cancer, a larger proportion of cases of invasive disease can be expected because relapse occurs in approximately half the patients with superficial disease and in many of these is associated with invasion of the bladder wall.

The management of invasive bladder carcinoma remains controversial, with no clear consensus about the optimal local treatment modality or about the role of associated or adjunctive systemic treatment. The choice of treatment is influenced more by physician bias, specialty training and geographical location than by the published results of clinical trials (Moore *et al*, 1988). Although radical cystectomy is currently regarded in North America as the standard management of muscle invasive disease, more than 50% of these patients will eventually relapse if treated with surgery alone. Similarly radiotherapy, which has been used more often in Britain, Australia and some parts of Europe, is also associated with relapses in more than 50% of cases. In both instances, recurrences are often associated with distant metastases, which has led to the use of systemic

*Present address: USC Norris Cancer Center, 1441 Eastlake Avenue, Los Angeles, California 90033

chemotherapy in association with local treatment approaches in an attempt to improve prognosis.

RADIOTHERAPY

Radiotherapy is rarely used alone for medically fit patients with invasive carcinoma of the bladder in the United States but is still commonly used in Canada and in Europe. However, in the United States radiotherapy is usually used as the treatment of choice for patients deemed unfit for surgery, introducing a clear patient selection bias when the outcomes of the two treatments are compared in a non-randomized fashion. Doses of external beam radiation have varied from 50 to 75 Gy, a better level of local tumour control being reported at the higher dosage range (Raghavan et al, 1997). There is no absolute consensus regarding field selection and field size, but there is general agreement that the whole pelvis should receive approximately 50–55 Gy, with a boost to the tumour of an additional 20 Gy. On the basis of several large series of cases of invasive bladder cancer (Bloom et al, 1982; Shipley et al, 1985; Gospodarowicz et al, 1989; Pollack et al, 1994; Mamegan et al, 1995), prognostic factors have been identified in patients treated with primary radiotherapy, including tumour grade, stage, tumour configuration, presence of carcinoma-in-situ, multifocal involvement, clinical complete remission after radiotherapy, transurethral resection of the tumour, presence of hydronephrosis, anaemia, dosage of irradiation and, in some series, the patient's age. Radiation therapy as a single modality achieves local control in 30–50% of patients with muscle invasive bladder cancer (Bloom et al, 1982; Shipley et al, 1985; Gospodarowicz et al, 1989; Pollack et al, 1994; Mamegan et al, 1995). However the 5 year survival of these patients is only 20–40%, depending on the prognostic factors listed above.

In the past, preoperative radiotherapy was investigated for localized muscle invasive bladder cancer in an attempt to improve the level of local control and thus to reduce the risk of dissemination (Bloom et al, 1982; Sell et al, 1991). The rationale behind such an approach was to downstage the tumour and improve "resectability" as well as to reduce the frequency of local recurrences. Although some trials suggested improved local control through this approach, there was no survival advantage in randomized trials when preoperative radiation followed by cystectomy was compared with radiotherapy alone (followed by salvage cystectomy in event of recurrence). In addition, the incidence of metastases was found to be similar in both groups. Preoperative radiotherapy therefore has largely lost favour despite its impact on local control (Cole et al, 1995). As a consequence, other strategies have been explored, most commonly the combination of cytotoxic chemotherapy with modalities of local tumour control, in an attempt to target both the primary tumour and occult metastases that may be present at first presentation. Three major approaches have been investigated, predicated on different timing—the use of chemotherapy during the period of radiotherapy, or alternatively before or after completion of local treatment.

CONCURRENT CHEMORADIATION

In many tumour types, extensive preclinical and clinical studies have shown that some cytotoxic agents, such as doxorubicin, cisplatin, carboplatin, 5-fluorouracil and mitomycin, exhibit radiosensitization, altering the response of tumour cells to the cytotoxic effects of radiation. It was thus logical that this strategy should be applied to the management of invasive bladder cancer. To date, most of the available data have been gleaned from phase I and II, non-randomized trials, and it is thus difficult to determine the true usefulness of this approach. It is clear that at least 50% of tumours are downstaged by concurrent chemotherapy and radiotherapy, but the impact on survival (compared with radiotherapy alone) is difficult to discern because of many factors, such as case selection bias, stage migration and changes in protocols of treatment delivery. Several of these studies are summarized in Table 1 (Housset *et al*, 1993; Kaufman *et al*, 1993; Tester *et al*, 1993; Dunst *et al*, 1994; Coppin *et al*, 1996).

One of the most important studies of chemoradiation for invasive bladder cancer was reported by the National Cancer Institute of Canada (Coppin *et al*, 1996). In this prospective, multicentre randomized trial, 99 patients were assigned to receive treatment with preoperative radiotherapy followed by cystectomy or radiotherapy alone as definitive local therapy, according to the preferences of the patients or the treating clinicians. These patients were then randomly allocated to receive cisplatin concurrently with radiation or radiation without chemotherapy. Improved local control was achieved with concurrent chemotherapy but without any difference in survival in the two groups (Coppin *et al*, 1996). However, an important potential bias was introduced by the selection process for definitive local therapy, and the study was marred by the small number of cases. In fact, the absence of survival benefit may have been due simply to the fact that fewer than 30 cases had been followed for 5 years at the time of reporting, thus reducing the power to detect a small, but important, difference in survival.

An emphasis in the chemoradiotherapy trials has been bladder preservation, a concept that had an even greater importance before the development of surgical techniques for bladder reconstruction after cystectomy. The investigators

TABLE 1 Chemoradiation for invasive bladder cancer[a]

Series	No of patients	T stage	Salvage cystectomy	Overall survival	Median follow-up
Coppin *et al*, 1996	42	2-4	not applicable	61%/2 y	50 mo
Dunst *et al*, 1994	139	1-3	–	40%/7 y	12 mo
Housset *et al*, 1993	54	2-4	22%	59%/3 y	18–58 mo
Kaufmann *et al*, 1993	53	2-4	15%	53%/4 y	48 mo
Chauvet *et al*, 1996	109	2-4	28%	42%/3.5 y	55 mo
Tester *et al*, 1996	91	2-4	40%	62%/4 y	>48 mo

[a]Modified from Javle and Raghavan (1996)

at the Massachusetts General Hospital have carried out pioneering phase II trials to develop the concept of increasing the level of bladder preservation through concurrent chemoradiation (Kaufman *et al*, 1993). Their approach has been predicated on the use of extensive transurethral resection, followed by chemoradiotherapy and endoscopic reassessment after the delivery of 40 Gy. Patients with incomplete response and who are suitable for surgery have undergone radical cystectomy. Those with a complete response and those deemed unfit for surgery have continued treatment to radical doses of irradiation. With this strategy 45% of a series of 53 patients with stages T_2–T_4 disease were alive and free of disease with a median follow-up of 4 years.

Similarly the Radiation Therapy Oncology Group (RTOG) has assessed the use of chemoradiation, initially with cisplatin as radiosensitizer (Dunst *et al*, 1994), demonstrating an acceptable profile of activity and toxicity. The RTOG (Tester *et al*, 1996) has also recently published the results of a phase II study in which 91 eligible patients with stages T_2–T_{4a} invasive bladder cancer were treated with two courses of methotrexate, cisplatin and vinblastine (MCV) followed by radiotherapy and concurrent cisplatin. The group reported a 43% risk of local failure, 22% risk of metastases and an overall survival of 42% with a 44% actuarial survival with an intact bladder at a median follow-up of 4 years. These results indicate that bladder preservation is possible in a select group of patients, especially those with a good performance status and node negative stages T_2–T_{4a} disease.

These investigators have taken the view that there is no requirement to confirm a survival benefit from chemoradiation per se, provided that statistically significant improvement in local control is achieved by this approach (as has been demonstrated by Coppin *et al*, 1996). Their view is that systemic therapy or some other strategy will be required to achieve a survival benefit, because invasive bladder cancer is a systemic disease at first presentation.

For completeness, it should be noted that an analogous approach to chemoradiotherapy has been taken in two trials of perioperative chemotherapy for invasive bladder cancer. The Eastern Cooperative Oncology Group administered the combination of methotrexate, vinblastine, doxorubicin and cisplatin (MVAC) before and after cystectomy, and demonstrated that the approach is feasible (Dreicer *et al*, 1990). However, despite the fact that this was not a randomized trial, there was no suggestion of a major improvement in outcome from this strategy, the complete remission rate being a modest 30%.

Similarly, Logothetis *et al* (1996) reported a randomized trial that was purportedly a comparison between neoadjuvant and adjuvant MVAC chemotherapy in patients undergoing cystectomy. As has been discussed in detail elsewhere (Raghavan, 1996a), this trial actually compared perioperative chemotherapy with classical adjuvant chemotherapy, and at the time of reporting did not show a survival benefit from either approach.

In view of the similarity of timing of systemic chemotherapy in relation to the definitive local treatment, these trials can be viewed as analogous to the strategy of chemoradiation, at least with respect to the attempt to improve overall survival by control of occult metastases.

SYSTEMIC CHEMOTHERAPY FOR INVASIVE BLADDER CANCER

It has long been believed that foci of micrometastases are present at the time of initial presentation of invasive bladder cancer, providing another reason for the addition of systemic chemotherapy to locoregional treatment in an attempt to improve cure rates. Most of the early information on chemotherapy for invasive bladder cancer was derived from the trials in metastatic disease. Cisplatin was reported as the most active single agent with a response rate of 20–30% in phase II and III studies (Raghavan *et al*, 1997). A variety of other agents have similar anticancer activity, including cyclophosphamide, the vinca alkaloids, methotrexate, 5-fluorouracil, doxorubicin, mitomycin C and, more recently, paclitaxel, gemcitabine, ifosphamide and gallium nitrate. Combination chemotherapy has been the mainstay of treatment of advanced bladder cancer since an Intergroup trial revealed a small but statistically significant survival advantage from the use of the MVAC regimen, compared with single agent cisplatin alone (Loehrer *et al*, 1992). Long term follow-up in this study revealed that 17% of patients receiving combination therapy were alive at 5 years, whereas there were few survivors in the single agent cisplatin arm (Saxman *et al*, 1997). This confirmed the role of the MVAC regimen but also illustrated the continuing need for more active treatment regimens.

Neoadjuvant Chemotherapy

Neoadjuvant or pre-emptive chemotherapy is the strategy of treatment in which systemic chemotherapy is given initially in the hope of downstaging the tumour, with an increased potential for resection, and with the potential for in vivo assessment of tumour response and possible radiosensitization. On the other hand it may delay potentially curative locally directed treatment.

Most single arm studies using this approach have shown substantial tumour downstaging, but have not been designed to assess potential survival advantage (Raghavan, 1991). A recent meta-analysis of all known randomized trials, reviewing information on 479 cases comparing local therapy alone with neoadjuvant chemotherapy followed by local treatment, demonstrated a 2% increase in relative risk of death with neoadjuvant therapy and an overall hazard ratio of 1.02 favouring local treatment alone (Ghersi *et al*, 1995). It should be emphasized that this study was dominated by studies that employed single agent chemotherapy regimens and has been criticized on the basis that the systemic treatment was not optimal.

Consequent upon the demonstration of the utility of the MVAC regimen for metastatic disease, Scher and colleagues applied this treatment in the neoadjuvant setting and recorded impressive tumour downstaging in patients with locally advanced disease (Scher *et al*, 1989). Several other non-randomized phase II studies also suggested similar results from aggressive combination chemotherapy schedules (Sternberg *et al*, 1993; Vogelzang *et al*, 1993; Srougi and Simon, 1994). However, a cautionary note was sounded by the mature follow-up data from the Memorial Sloan Kettering Cancer Center, New York, in which the early results (Scher *et al*, 1989) did not translate into an apparent increase in long term survival and were marred by a high rate of local and distant relapse (Schultz *et al*, 1994).

In a large international study, undertaken by the European Organization for the Research and Treatment of Cancer (EORTC), the UK Medical Research Council (MRC), and several other national groups, nearly 1000 patients were randomly allocated to receive neoadjuvant cisplatin, methotrexate and vinblastine (CMV regimen) plus local therapy or local therapy alone (Hall, 1996). The preliminary report supports the result of the above meta-analysis, with a failure to reveal any significant survival difference between the two arms.

However, one important randomized study, performed by the Nordic Cooperative Bladder Cancer Study Group, did reveal a statistically significant survival benefit from neoadjuvant chemotherapy (Malmstrom *et al*, 1996). In this trial, 325 patients with invasive bladder cancer were allocated to treatment with cystectomy or neoadjuvant doxorubicin plus cisplatin followed by cystectomy. After 5 years, the overall survival was 59% in the combined modality group and 51% in the cystectomy group. There was a statistically significant difference in survival for patients with T_3–T_4 disease.

Another important randomized trial, conducted by the North American Intergroup, has yet to be reported. In this study, a target of more than 300 patients will be randomly allocated to radical cystectomy or to neoadjuvant MVAC chemotherapy followed by cystectomy. If this trial fails to show an overall survival impact of chemotherapy, it would be reasonable to abandon this strategy. However, if a survival benefit is demonstrated, neoadjuvant chemotherapy will have to be viewed as one of the new standards of therapy. Although the results of the EORTC/MRC study are compelling, it is not without flaws, and the absence of survival benefit could be explained by such factors as a large number of treating centres, absence of central histological review, and potentially variable implementation of the study protocol in different centres.

Adjuvant Chemotherapy

Like the rationale for the use of neoadjuvant chemotherapy, the strategy of adjuvant administration of cytotoxics is based on the observation that most relapses after locoregional treatment for invasive bladder cancer are associated with distant metastases. The principal disadvantage of adjuvant chemotherapy is that response cannot be assessed directly, and there is thus no way of knowing prospectively whether the treatment is having any beneficial impact. Furthermore, as the response rate of even the most active combination regi-

TABLE 2. Randomized trials of adjuvant chemotherapy for bladder cancer

Series	Stage	No of patients	Primary therapy	Chemotherapy	Survival	Reference
USC 1991	T3b-T4, NX, M0	91	Cystectomy	CAP Observation	70%/3 y 46%	Skinner et al, 1991
Mainz 1992	T3b-T4a, N+, M0	49	Cystectomy	MVAC Observation	63%/3 y 0	Stockle et al, 1992
SAKK 1994	Ta-4, N+, M0	77	Cystectomy	Cisplatin Observation	57%/5 y 54%	Studer et al, 1994
Stanford 1995	T3b-T4, N+, M0	55	Cystectomy	CMV Observation	40%/5 y 38%	Freiha et al, 1996

Mainz = University of Mainz; SAKK = Swiss Cooperative Cancer Group; Stanford = Stanford University; USC = University of Southern California

mens is only about 65%, many patients will be treated without likely benefit. By contrast, it should not be forgotten that randomized trials have validated the role of adjuvant chemotherapy for node-positive breast cancer, despite an equivalently active set of systemic therapies.

Four randomized trials of adjuvant chemotherapy following radical primary therapy have been reported (Skinner et al, 1991; Stockle et al, 1992; Studer et al, 1994; Freiha et al, 1996) (Table 2). In each instance, the adjuvant treatment was administered after cystectomy. We are unaware of any randomized trials that have assessed the impact of adjuvant chemotherapy after completion of definitive radiotherapy for invasive bladder cancer.

At the University of Southern California, 91 patients with P_3–P_4 or node positive bladder cancer were randomly allocated after cystectomy to observation or adjuvant chemotherapy with cyclophosphamide, doxorubicin and cisplatin (CAP regimen) (Skinner et al, 1991). In a somewhat controversial report, Skinner and colleagues reported significant differences in disease free and total survival favouring the adjuvant chemotherapy group. However, since the number of cases was relatively small and because treatment was modified on the basis of soft agar clonogenic assay testing, the accuracy and validity of the study have been questioned.

Several randomized trials have failed to show any survival benefit from CAP chemotherapy over single agent cisplatin for metastatic disease (Raghavan et al, 1990). Furthermore, analogous to the Intergroup trial that demonstrated the superiority of the MVAC regimen over single agent cisplatin, Logothetis et al have shown that the MVAC regimen confers improved survival compared with the CAP regimen for patients with advanced bladder cancer (Logothetis et al, 1990). It is thus not surprising that Studer and colleagues, reporting the results of a randomized study of a Swiss collaborative group, were unable to show a survival impact of adjuvant single agent cisplatin after cystectomy (Stadler et al, in press) and that the CAP regimen also had little impact as adjuvant therapy (Skinner et al, 1991).

However, Stockle and colleagues have reported a statistically significant increase in disease free survival from the use of adjuvant MVEC chemotherapy (with epirubicin replacing doxorubicin) after cystectomy for high stage/node positive bladder cancer, compared with the outcome of cystectomy alone (Stockle *et al*, 1992). This trial was closed prematurely when it was recognized that the trial design, which precluded the use of salvage chemotherapy for relapsing patients, was potentially causing a significant reduction in survival in the control patients. As implemented, this study confirms the benefits of chemotherapy at some time after cystectomy, rather than validating the role of classical adjuvant therapy. Furthermore, because of the necessary early closure, this study is underpowered, and the confidence intervals of the outcomes are very wide.

At Stanford University (Freiha *et al*, 1996), in a study intended to resolve the question above, 55 patients with pathological stage T_{3b} and T_4 tumours or pelvic lymph node involvement were randomized to treatment with CMV or observation after cystectomy. Patients in the observation arm were offered the same chemotherapy at time of relapse, thus allowing a true test of the role of early adjuvant chemotherapy. With a median follow-up of 62 months, the time to progression in patients treated with CMV adjuvant therapy was significantly longer than in the observation group (median 37 versus 12 months). However, the overall survival in the two groups was not statistically significantly different, with a trend favouring the adjuvant chemotherapy group. This can be explained by the high rate of salvage by chemotherapy in relapsed patients in the observation arm and by the very small number of cases for a randomized trial. Also of relevance, Wei *et al*, reporting experience of patients treated in Taiwan with cystectomy and adjuvant CMV chemotherapy, have documented a disturbingly high relapse rate, sounding an important note of caution (Wei *et al*, 1996). Thus these studies suggest an improved disease free survival among patients treated with adjuvant chemotherapy but without a clear impact on overall survival, and it would be premature to regard adjuvant chemotherapy as constituting any established standard of care.

FUTURE PROSPECTS

There has been important recent progress in two aspects of the management of bladder cancer which may have an impact on the use of combined modality treatment for invasive disease. As noted above, several promising new agents have been shown to have activity against advanced bladder cancer. Paclitaxel, derived from the bark of the Pacific yew tree, inhibits microtubule assembly, among other functions. This agent has been shown to have substantial activity against bladder cancer (Roth *et al*, 1994), as well as being a potent radiosensitizer.

Gemcitabine, a fluorinated derivative of cytosine arabinoside, which has a greater level of intracellular uptake and retention than the parent compound, has recently been shown to be highly active against bladder cancer, both previously treated and untreated (Pollera *et al*, 1994; Stadler *et al*, in press). This agent also is a known radiosensitizer.

A hybrid agent, AD-312, which combines the functions of an anthracycline and a nitrosourea, has been shown in our laboratory to be active against doxorubicin resistant and cisplatin resistant bladder cancer xenografts (Glaves *et al*, 1996). This agent also has the potential to function as a radiosensitizer.

Each of these novel compounds has the potential to allow a new level of interaction between systemic chemotherapy and local radiation, although the morbidity caused by AD-312 is not yet known. Both paclitaxel and gemcitabine are well tolerated by elderly patients, which may allow greater flexibility for their use as preoperative or pre-radiotherapy neoadjuvant regimens, or may even facilitate a less toxic approach to adjuvant chemotherapy.

In addition to the progress in the development of novel cytotoxic compounds, there is an increased understanding of the molecular determinants of prognosis and of response to treatment (Raghavan, 1996b). For example there is now clear evidence of the presence of apoptotic markers in response to radiotherapy for bladder cancer, which may allow earlier determination of the likely outcome of treatment (Chyle *et al*, 1996). The epidermal growth factor (EGF) receptor has an established function as a prognostic determinant of the natural history of bladder cancer; and there is now preclinical evidence that the interplay between EGF and its receptor may predict response to cisplatin and other cytotoxic agents (Christen *et al*, 1990; Fan *et al*, 1993), although this has not been confirmed in clinical studies of bladder cancer. In addition, we have shown, in a series of xenografts and human biopsy specimens of bladder cancer, very high levels of expression of glutathione, an intracellular scavenger of cisplatin and other cytotoxics (Pendyala *et al*, 1997). In other tumour types, depletion of intracellular glutathione has led to enhanced sensitivity to chemotherapy, although this has not yet been tested in bladder cancer.

Our increased understanding of these concepts, augmented by the availability of active novel compounds with radiosensitizing potential, suggests that important progress will soon be made. In order to maximize the rate of change, scientific method and carefully structured clinical trials must continue to govern our investigations.

SUMMARY

Invasive bladder cancer is associated with locoregional and distant metastases. To improve the outcome of management, systemic chemotherapy has been combined with locoregional treatment. Programmes have been structured in which chemotherapy is administered before or after definitive radiotherapy or surgery, or in combination with radiotherapy. Most randomized trials to date have failed to define a survival benefit from initial chemotherapy, but evidence is emerging that classical adjuvant chemotherapy may improve survival. New cytotoxic agents, including paclitaxel and gemcitabine, accompanied by an emerging understanding of the factors governing cytotoxic drug resistance, may also lead to better management.

References

Bloom HJG, Hendry WF, Wallace DM and Skeet RG (1982) Treatment of T3 bladder cancer: controlled trial of preoperative radiotherapy and radical cystectomy versus radical radiotherapy. Second report and review. *British Journal of Urology* **54** 136–151

Chauvet B, Brewer Y, Felix-Faure C, Davin J-L, Choquenet C and Reboul F (1996) Concurrent cisplatin and radiotherapy for patients with muscle invasive bladder cancer who are not candidates for radical cystectomy. *Journal of Urology* **156** 1258–1262

Christen RD, Hom DK, Porter DC *et al* (1990) Epidermal growth factor regulates the in vitro sensitivity of human ovarian carcinoma cells to cisplatin. *Journal of Clinical Investigation* **86** 1632–1640

Chyle V, Pollack A, Czerniak B *et al* (1996) Apoptosis and downstaging after preoperative radiotherapy for muscle-invasive bladder cancer. *International Journal of Oncology, Biology, Physics* **35** 281–287

Cole CJ, Pollack A, Zagars GK *et al* (1995) Local control of muscle invasive bladder cancer: preoperative radiotherapy and cystectomy versus cystectomy alone. *International Journal of Radiation Oncology, Biology, Physics* **32** 331–340

Coppin CML, Gospodarowicz MK, James K *et al* (1996) Improved local control of invasive bladder cancer by concurrent cisplatin and preoperative or definitive radiation. *Journal of Clinical Oncology* **14** 2901–2907

Dreicer R, Messing EM, Loehrer PJ and Trump DL (1990) Perioperative methotrexate, vinblastine, doxorubicin and cisplatin (MVAC) for poor risk transitional carcinoma of the bladder: an Eastern Cooperative Oncology Group pilot study. *Journal of Urology* **144** 1123–1127

Dunst J, Sauer R, Schrott KM *et al* (1994) Organ-sparing treatment of advanced bladder cancer: a 10-year experience. *International Journal of Radiation Oncology, Biology, Physics* **30** 261–266

Fan Z, Baselga J, Masui H and Mendelsohn J (1993) Antitumor effect of anti-epidermal growth factor receptor monoclonal antibodies plus cis-diammine-dichloroplatinum on well established A431 cell xenografts. *Cancer Research* **53** 4637–4642

Freiha F, Reese J and Torti FM (1996) A randomized trial of radical cystectomy plus cisplatin, vinblastine and methotrexate chemotherapy for muscle invasive bladder cancer. *Journal of Urology* **155** 495–500

Ghersi D, Stewart LA, Parmar MKB et al (1995) Does neoadjuvant cisplatin based chemotherapy improve survival of patients with locally advanced bladder cancer? A meta analysis of individual patient data from randomized clinical trials. *Journal of Urology* **75** 206–213

Glaves D, Murray M, Raghavan D (1996) Novel bifunctional anthracycline and nitrosourea chemotherapy for human bladder cancer: analysis in a preclinical survival model. *Clinical Cancer Research* **2** 1315–1319

Gospodarowicz MK, Hawkins NV, Rawlings GA et al (1989) Radical radiotherapy for muscle invasive transitional cell carcinoma of the bladder: failure analysis. *Journal of Urology* **142** 1448–1454

Hall RR (1996) Neo-adjuvant CMV chemotherapy and cystectomy or radiotherapy in muscle invasive bladder cancer: first analysis of MRC/EORTC intercontinental trial. *Proceedings of the American Society for Clinical Oncology* **15** 244

Housset M, Maulard C, Chretien Y et al (1993) Combined radiation and chemotherapy for invasive transitional cell carcinoma of the bladder: a prospective study. *Journal of Clinical Oncology* **11** 2150–2157

Javle M and Raghavan D (1996) Systemic chemotherapy for invasive bladder cancer. *Cancer*

Control **3** 501–506

Kaufman, DS, Shipley WU, Griffin PP *et al* (1993) Selective bladder preservation by combination treatment of invasive bladder cancer. *New England Journal of Medicine* **329** 1377–1382

Loehrer PJ, Einhorn LH, Elson PJ *et al* (1992) A randomized comparison of cisplatin alone or in combination with methotrexate, vinblastine and doxorubicin in patients with metastatic urothelial carcinoma. *Journal of Clinical Oncology* **10** 1066–1073

Logothetis, CJ, Dexeus FH, Finn L *et al* (1990) A prospective randomised trial comparing MVAC and CISCA chemotherapy for patients with metastatic urothelial tumors. *Journal of Clinical Oncology* **8** 1050–1055

Logothetis CJ, Swanson D, Amato R *et al* (1996) Optimal delivery of perioperative chemotherapy: preliminary results of a randomized, prospective, comparative trial of preoperative and postoperative chemotherapy for invasive bladder carcinoma. *Journal of Urology* **155** 1241–1245

Malmstrom P-U, Rintal E, Wahlqvist R *et al* (1996) Five-year followup of a prospective trial of radical cystectomy and neoadjuvant chemotherapy: Nordic Cystectomy Trial I. *Journal of Urology* **155** 1903–1906

Mameghan H, Fisher R, Mameghan J and Brook S (1995) Analysis of failure following definitive radiotherapy for invasive transitional cell carcinoma of the bladder. *International Journal of Radiation Oncology, Biology, Physics* **31** 247–254

Moore MJ, O'Sullivan B and Tannock IF (1988) How expert physicians would wish to be treated if they had genitourinary cancer. *Journal of Clinical Oncology* **6** 1736–1745

Pendyala L, Raghavan D, Velagapudi S *et al* (1997) Translational studies of glutathione in bladder cancer cell lines and human specimens. *Clinical Cancer Research* **3** 793–798

Pollack A, Zagars GK and Swanson DA (1994) Muscle invasive bladder cancer treated with external beam radiotherapy: prognostic factors. *International Journal of Radiation Oncology, Biology, Physics* **30** 267–277

Pollera CF, Ceribelli A, Crecco M and Calabresi F (1994) Weekly gemcitabine in advanced bladder cancer: a preliminary report. *Annals of Oncology* **5** 132–134

Raghavan D (1991) A critical assessment of trials of neoadjuvant (preemptive) chemotherapy for bladder cancer: lesson for future studies of combined modality treatment. *International Journal of Radiation Oncology, Biology, Physics* **20** 233–237

Raghavan D (1996a) Editorial: perioperative chemotherapy for invasive bladder cancer—what should we tell our patients? *Journal of Urology* **155** 1246–1247

Raghavan D (1996b) Are Voltaire, Rousseau et al finally wrong? *Lancet* **348** 17

Raghavan D, Shipley WU, Garnick MB, Russell PJ and Richie JP (1990) Biology and management of bladder cancer. *New England Journal of Medicine* **322** 1129–1138

Raghavan D, Shipley WU, Hall RR and Richie JP (1997) Biology and management of invasive bladder cancer, In: Raghavan D, Scher HI, Leibel SA and Lange PH (eds). *Principles and Practice of Genitourinary Oncology*, pp 281–298, Lippincott-Raven Publishers, Philadelphia

Roth BJ, Dreicer R, Einhorn LH *et al* (1994) Significant activity of paclitaxel in advanced transitional cell carcinoma of the urothelium: a phase II trial of the Eastern Cooperative Oncology Group. *Journal of Clinical Oncology* **12** 2264–2270

Saxman SB, Propert K, Einhorn LH *et al* (1997) Long term follow up of phase III intergroup study of cisplatin alone or in combination with methotrexate, vinblastine and doxorubicin in patients with metastatic urothelial carcinoma. *Journal of Clinical Oncology* **15** 2564–2569

Scher H, Herr H, Sternberg C *et al* (1989) Neo-adjuvant chemotherapy for invasive bladder cancer: experience with the M-VAC regimen. *British Journal of Urology* **64** 250–256

Schultz PK, Herr HW, Zhang Z-F *et al* (1994) Neoadjuvant chemotherapy for invasive bladder cancer: prognostic factors for survival of patients treated with M-VAC with 5-year follow-up. *Journal of Clinical Oncology* **12** 1394–1401

Sell A, Jakobsen A and Nostrom B (1991) Treatment of advanced bladder cancer category T_2, T_3, T_{4a}. *Scandinavian Journal of Urology and Nephrology—Supplement* **138** 193–201

Shipley WU, Rose MA, Perrone TL *et al* (1985) Full-dose irradiation for patients with invasive bladder carcinoma: clinical and histological factors prognostic of improved survival. *Journal of Urology* **134** 679–683

Skinner DG, Daniels JR, Russell CA *et al* (1991) The role of adjuvant chemotherapy following cystectomy for invasive bladder cancer: a prospective comparative trial. *Journal of Urology* **145** 459–467

Srougi M and Simon SD (1994) Primary methotrexate, vinblastine, doxorubicin and cisplatin chemotherapy and bladder preservation in locally invasive bladder cancer: a 5-year followup. *Journal of Urology* **151** 593–597

Stadler W, Kuzel T, Raghavan D *et al* Phase II trial of gemcitabine for advanced bladder cancer. *Journal of Clinical Oncology* (in press)

Sternberg CN, Arena MG, Calabresi F *et al* (1993) Neoadjuvant M-VAC (methotrexate, vinblastine, doxorubicin and cisplatin) for infiltrating transitional cell carcinoma of the bladder. *Cancer* **72** 1975–1982

Stockle M, Meyenburg W, Wellek S *et al* (1992) Advanced bladder cancer (stages pT_{3b}, pT_{4a}, pN_1 and pN_2): improved survival after radical cystectomy and 3 adjuvant cycles of chemotherapy: results of a controlled prospective study. *Journal of Urology* **148** 302–307

Studer UE, Bacchi M, Biedermann C *et al* (1994) Adjuvant cisplatin chemotherapy following cystectomy for bladder cancer: results of a prospective randomized trial. *Journal of Urology* **152** 81–84

Tester W, Porter A, Asbell S *et al* (1993) Combined modality program with possible organ preservation for invasive bladder carcinoma: results of RTOG protocol 85–12. *International Journal of Radiation Oncology, Biology, Physics* **25** 783–790

Tester W, Caplan R, Heaney J *et al* (1996) Neoadjuvant combined modality program with selective organ preservation for invasive bladder cancer: results of Radiation Therapy Oncology Group phase II trial 8802. *Journal of Clinical Oncology* **14** 119–127

Vogelzang NJ, Moormeier JA, Awan AM *et al* (1993) Methotrexate, vinblastine, doxorubicin and cisplatin followed by radiotherapy or surgery for muscle invasive bladder cancer: the University of Chicago experience. *Journal of Urology* **149** 753–757

Wei C-H, Hsieh R-K, Chiou T-J *et al* (1996) Adjuvant methotrexate, vinblastine and cisplatin chemotherapy for invasive transitional cell carcinoma: Taiwan experience. *Journal of Urology* **155** 118–121

The authors are responsible for the accuracy of the references.

Future Directions

MALCOLM J COPTCOAT[1] • R T D OLIVER[2]

[1]*Department of Urology, King's College Hospital, London SE5 9RS;*[2]*Department of Medical Oncology, St Bartholomew's Hospital, London EC1A 7BE*

That there has been no major improvement over the past 20 years in the chances of cure for a patient presenting with bladder cancer is not an unreasonable conclusion of this review. There is, however, a fresh sense of optimism that with new drugs and a better understanding of timing to maximize the benefits from multimodality therapy as well new understanding of the biology, there is considerable potential to be gained from reappraising this tumour. At the practical clinical level, there can be little doubt that one area of remarkable progress has been in the design of continent bladder reconstruction. This procedure is very impressive when it is successful, leading to its use earlier in the natural history, reducing the risks from clonal diversification and development of local invasion and metastases. However, the need for further surgery in a minority of patients means that there remains room for improvement.

From a scientific perspective, there has been major progress in understanding clonal development, even though bladder cancer has not had quite the funding priority of breast, prostate and bowel cancer. With easy access for repeated samples of tumour tissue, through urine cytology and cystoscopy, and the long natural history of the disease, bladder cancer offers considerable opportunity for understanding the progress of clonal development of cancer. Pathologically, even in the conventional transitional cell cancers in the west, more attention needs to be paid to the issue of squamous metaplasia. With better morphology and new techniques such as the dot enzyme linked immunosorbent assay this is being recognized more frequently than previously. That there needs to be greater awareness among clinicians that clonal evolution is an active ongoing process is highlighted by Lightman and Droller's chapter that demonstrates the impact of smoking intensity on increasing grade and extent of invasion in bladder tumours.

With similar data coming from study of melanoma, breast, prostate and testis cancer, cancers whose induction is not normally associated with smoking, it does seem that this issue is of general interest in understanding clonal development of cancer. As there are data from our own studies showing a higher intensity of smoking among bladder cancer patients with metastases and those with recurrent superficial cancer who relapse early after BCG induced remission, there is a clear need to focus urologists' attention on this issue. That there are still patients followed for many years in cystoscopy clinics who continue smoking without any encouragement to stop and present 5–10 years later with advanced disease is something that needs to be highlighted.

It is possible that greater attention to the issue of squamous metaplasia will make its greatest impact in the area of understanding papillomavirus involvement in bladder cancer. The recognition from study of the role of bovine papillomavirus in cattle bladder cancer, which highlights the need for squamous change to facilitate viral replication, and more significantly how the virus may play a hit and run role in tumour initiation that is blocked by vaccination, provides an excellent background for understanding the fact that less than 20% of tumours have evidence of virus detectable and in these patients it is as often in normal tissue as in tumour tissue.

The exciting progress that has been made in understanding the cytogenetic changes in clonal development, particularly in understanding chromosomes 9 and 17, is highlighted by Knowles's chapter. However, the need to do more detailed molecular studies on these tumours is highlighted by the progress in the cattle bovine papillomavirus model and study of human papillomavirus induced cervix cancer, where there are differences between viral positive and negative tumours in terms of molecular changes. The potential of some of the tumour membrane changes, such as expression of epidermal growth factor receptor and tumour angiogenesis as therapeutic targets in the most malignant life threatening subtypes of bladder cancer, is highlighted in the chapter by Neil and provides tantalizing opportunities for the future.

For the time being in terms of the greatest gain for the largest proportion of bladder cancer, focusing on use of immune manipulation with BCG or keyhole limpet haemocyanin is likely to be a more productive area, as emphasized by Lamm. With the recognition that this disease has a 10–20 year potential natural history, it is clear that better understanding and more trials will need to be focused on aspects of remission maintenance. This could also be a fruitful area for scientific endeavour, given the evidence from animal models and cervix cancer that different alleles in HLA class II, possibly mediated via linkage to immune response regulating genes, have an important role in determining susceptibility to resistance to papillomavirus.

The importance of major histocompatibility antigen loss as an immune escape mechanism and, more significantly, its correction by gene therapy, offers a major hope for development of in vivo gene therapy, given the animal models showing its ability to induce bystander immunity. Bladder cancer, because of its ease of access and long natural history, will be a particularly good tumour in which to study this approach. However, these studies will only succeed if urologists recognize their central role in ensuring that tumour tissue is harvested in a form suitable for molecular studies. Although these primarily use whole tissue for DNA extraction, which of necessity disrupts tumour architecture, DNA in situ techniques are improving. The need for frozen, in addition to formalin fixed tissue banks, as well as better usage of urine exfoliated cells from bladder washings for culture studies will be critical for the future. Urologists will also need to focus on developing and improving their skills in monitoring and documenting digitally the response of local disease to treatment. This will be in addition to the understandable interest in becoming competent at bladder reconstruction. The results of these operations will only improve if the urologist has a sufficient referral practice to do the operation frequently.

Though there has been a tendency to forget the value of chemotherapy and radiation treatment because surgical reconstruction is so much more difficult after treatment, the chapter by Raghavan reminds us how active modern treatments are in achieving durable complete remission and the increasing potential for exploration of synergy between radiation and chemotherapy. Furthermore, with the range of new agents and in particular encouraging early results from paclitaxel and gemcitabine these may completely alter attitudes to treatment. With more and more data highlighting the importance of a functioning *TP53* gene in determining success of both radiation and chemotherapy and the first successes of *TP53* gene therapy having been reported, it is to be hoped that there will be more progress in the clinical arena to report in 20 years' time than have emerged from the past 20 years.

Biographical Notes

Suhail Baithun, a graduate of Baghdad University, took the MRCPath in 1983. He is currently senior lecturer and honorary consultant in the department of morbid anatomy at the St Bartholomew's and Royal London Hospital School of Medicine and Dentistry, with a specialist interest in the pathology of urological cancers.

Judith Breuer graduated from the Middlesex Hospital Medical School in 1981 and obtained an MD from the National Institute of Medical Research in 1995. She is currently senior lecturer in virology at Queen Mary and Westfield College. Her main research interest is the molecular epidemiology of virus infections.

M Saveria Campo obtained her PhD in genetics at the University of Edinburgh. She joined the Beatson Institute for Cancer Research in Glasgow in 1981, where she is a senior group leader. Her work focuses on cell transformation by papillomavirus, immune response to viral infection and vaccine development. She is a Cancer Research Campaign life fellow and was awarded a professorship by Glasgow University in 1996.

Malcolm J Coptcoat is a senior lecturer in surgical oncology and honorary consultant urologist at King's College Hospital, London. He graduated from Liverpool University in 1979 and, following his training in general surgery and urology, now concentrates on the role of minimally invasive surgery in the treatment of urological malignancy.

Pallon Daruwala is currently a specialist training registrar in the department of urology, Dundee Royal Infirmary.

Michael J Droller, MD, is chairman of the department of urology at the Mount Sinai School of Medicine, New York. He received his medical degree from Harvard Medical School and his urological training at Stanford University Medical Center. Before his present appointment he was on the faculty at the Johns Hopkins School of Medicine for seven years. His primary interest is urological oncology, particularly the biology and clinical management of bladder cancer.

Miland Javle qualified in India, completed his training in internal medicine at the State University of New York and is currently a fellow in medical oncology at Roswell Park Cancer Institute. He has worked in the multidisciplinary genitourinary cancer clinic for the past two years and has published widely on the management of bladder and prostate cancer.

Margaret A Knowles, a graduate of Bristol University, received her PhD from the University of London for studies on in vitro transformation of epithelial cells carried out in the laboratory of Dr Leonard Franks at the Imperial Cancer Research Fund Laboratories. She is currently professor of experimental cancer research at the University of Leeds and deputy director of the ICRF Cancer Medicine Research Unit at St James' Hospital, Leeds. Her research interests focus on the identification of genes involved in development and progression of bladder cancer.

Donald L Lamm began immunotherapy studies of BCG in bladder cancer in animal models during his urology residency at the University of California, San Diego, in 1973. In 1980 he reported the first controlled clinical trial demonstrating the superiority of BCG over surgery alone. As principal investigator for the Southwest Oncology Group he has directed several clinical trials of BCG in the treatment of bladder cancer.

Jaime Landman, MD, an undergraduate at the University of Michigan and a medical student at the Columbia College of Physicians and Surgeons, is presently a urology resident at the Mount Sinai Medical Center, New York. He will be a fellow in endourology and laparoscopy at the Washington University School of Medicine in 1999.

John Lunec graduated in physics from Imperial College, London, in 1971 and obtained a PhD in biophysics. In 1986 he joined the cancer research unit at the University of Newcastle upon Tyne Medical School, where he is currently senior lecturer in molecular oncology, head of the molecular biology section and assistant director. His research interest is the molecular biology of cancer, focusing particularly on bladder and ovarian adult cancers and on paediatric neural tumours.

VH Nargund graduated from Karnatak University in 1981 and then undertook a research fellowship at the cancer research unit at the University of Bradford. He is currently working as a consultant urologist at St Bartholomew's Hospital, London.

David E Neal is professor of surgery and head of the school of surgical sciences in the University of Newcastle upon Tyne. His clinical and research interests are centred on urological oncology and reconstruction.

AME Nouri graduated from the University of London in 1979 with a BSc in immunology and gained his PhD in immunology in 1982. He undertook a project at Guy's Hospital, London, to investigate the involvement of cytokines in rheumatic diseases. He currently works at The Royal London Hospital with Professor Oliver in the department of medical oncology, investigating the role of gene therapy and immunotherapy in cancer.

RTD Oliver graduated from the University of Cambridge and The London Hospital in 1966. He undertook postgraduate research on HLA and transplantation immunology with Hilliard Festenstein and received an MD in 1974. He trained in oncology with Gordon Hamilton-Fairley at St Bartholomew's Hospital and in urology with John Blandy at St Peter's Hospital and the Institute of Urology. He is currently on the staff of The Royal Hospitals NHS Trust, is professor in medical oncology at Queen Mary & Westfield School of Medicine and runs a clinical research unit doing research in urological tumours.

Khaver N Qureshi qualified in medicine at the Medical College of St Bartholomew's Hospital in 1992 and obtained his FRCS in 1996. He is now working in the department of surgery and the cancer research unit, University of Newcastle upon Tyne, investigating the role of microsatellite alterations in bladder cancer.

Derek Raghavan is professor of medicine and urology at the University of Southern California, Los Angeles, chief of the division of medical oncology at USC and associate director for clinical research of the Norris Cancer Center. Until recently he was professor of medicine and urology at the State University of New York and chief of the departments of solid tumor oncology and investigational therapeutics at Roswell Park Cancer Institute, Buffalo, New York State. He has published more than 250 papers, books and chapters, predominantly on genitourinary cancer, lung cancer and the development of new anticancer agents.

Index

AAD-312, bladder cancer response, 157
Angiogenesis
    bladder cancer, 89–90
    clonal progression marker, 114
Aromatic amines, bladder cancer development, 7–8, 10–11
Artificial sweeteners, bladder cancer risk factor, 13

Bacille Calmette-Guérin (BCG). *See* Immunotherapy
BAX, expression in bladder cancer, 88
BCG. *See* Bacille Calmette-Guérin
BCL2, expression in bladder cancer, 88, 121–122
Bilharzia
    genetic alterations, 63–64
    incidence, 63
    screening, 23–24
    squamous bladder cancer promotion, 20–24, 63
    TP53 mutations, 24
Bladder reconstruction, 139–141
Bovine papillomavirus (BPV)
    bladder cancer association, 18, 20, 39–40
    classification, 39
    hit and run hypothesis, 25, 32–33
    immunosuppression in cancer development, 39–40
    oncogenesis mechanisms, 32–35
    vaccination in cancer control, 31, 43–44
BPV. *See* Bovine papillomavirus

Cadherin. *See* E-Cadherin
CAP regimen, bladder cancer response, 155
Carcinoma in situ (CIS)
    chemotherapy, 103–105
    culture, 135–136
    genetic alterations, 61–63, 67
    immunotherapy, 103
    progression, 66–67

transitional cell carcinoma comparison, 100–101
CCND1, amplification in bladder cancer, 53
CDKN1A, prognostic value, 87
CDKN2, alterations in bladder cancer, 54–55, 64, 82
Cell adhesion molecules, expression in bladder cancer, 90–91
Chemotherapy
    bladder cancer response and clinical studies, 3, 101, 103
    immunotherapy comparison, 99–100
    invasive bladder cancer
        adjuvant chemotherapy, 154–156
        chemoradiation, 151–153
        neoadjuvant chemotherapy, 153–154
        postsurgical therapy, 141–143
        TP53, sensitivity effects, 57, 92, 121, 163
Chromosome 9
    alterations in bladder cancer, 8–9, 53–55, 64–65, 67, 82, 110, 136
    screening for cancer, 24, 136
Chromosome 11p, alterations in bladder cancer, 83
Chromosome 13q, alterations in bladder cancer, 58, 83
Chromosome 17p, alterations in bladder cancer, 56–58, 65, 82, 110, 112
Cigarette smoking. *See* Smoking
CIS. *See* Carcinoma in situ
CMV regimen, bladder cancer response, 154, 156
Coffee, bladder cancer risk factor, 13

DCC, bladder cancer candidate gene, 83
DNA repair, defects in bladder cancer, 61

E5, oncogenesis mechanisms, 34–35
E6, oncogenesis mechanisms, 34
E7, oncogenesis mechanisms, 34

E-Cadherin, expression in bladder cancer, 90–91

EGFR. *See* Epidermal growth factor receptor

EMS1, amplification in bladder cancer, 53

Endoscopy, bladder cancer diagnosis, 133

Epidermal growth factor receptor (EGFR) gene in bladder cancer. *See ERBB2*
  prognostic value, 80–81, 92, 134, 137, 157
  structure, 80

Epidermodysplasia verruciformis, papillomavirus-associated cancers, 36–38

ERBB2, amplification and overexpression in bladder cancer, 53, 63, 81–82

FGF. *See* Fibroblast growth factor

Fibroblast growth factor (FGF), expression in bladder cancer, 89–90

G-CSF, expression in bladder cancer, 113

Gemcitabine, bladder cancer response, 156–157

Gender, bladder cancer distribution, 5, 17

Gene therapy
  approaches in bladder cancer, 143–144
  HLA-B7 gene therapy
    advanced cancer therapy with *TP53*, 120–122, 124–125
    early bladder cancer, rationale, 116–120
  TP53, 110, 120–122

Geographic epidemiology, 17

Glutathione *S*-transferase, deficiency in bladder cancer, 51

hCG. *See* Human chorionic gonadotropin

Heredity, bladder cancer, 51–52

HIV. *See* Human immunodeficiency virus

HLA
  class I expression correlation with ICAM1, 115–116
  HLA-B7 gene therapy
    advanced cancer therapy with *TP53*, 120–122, 124–125
    early bladder cancer, rationale, 116–120
  loss in escape from immune surveillance, 109–110, 115, 117
  prognostic value, 137

HPV. *See* Human papillomavirus

HSP70, expression in bladder cancer, 121–122

Human chorionic gonadotropin (hCG), squamous metaplasia expression, 19, 113–114, 137

Human immunodeficiency virus (HIV), papillomavirus-associated cancers, 35–36

Human papillomavirus (HPV)
  bladder cancer association, 18, 20, 30, 40–42, 162
  cancer types with infection, 22–23, 25, 29–31, 35–39
  cofactors in cancer deveopment, 29–30, 35–37, 41–42
  genome, 32
  hit and run hypothesis, 25, 32–33, 41
  oncogenesis mechanisms, 32–35
  screening bladder cancers, 42
  subtypes, 31–32
  vaccination in cancer control, 31, 42–44

ICAM1, HLA class I expression correlation, 115–116

Immunotherapy
  bacille Calmette-Guérin, 99–100, 103–105, 161–162
  carcinoma in situ, 103–105
  chemotherapy comparison, 99–100
  clinical trials, 103–105
  onset of action, 100
  smoking effects on response, 111–112, 161–162

Incidence, bladder cancer, 5

Interferon γ, HLA class I response, 116

Invasive bladder cancer
  chemoradiation, 151–153
  management overview, 149–150
  prognosis, 18
  progression, 12
  radiotherapy, 150, 156–157
  risk factors, 8–9, 12
  systemic chemotherapy
    adjuvant chemotherapy, 154–156
    neoadjuvant chemotherapy, 153–154

JUN, copy number in cancer, 80

LOH. *See* Loss of heterozygosity

Loss of heterozygosity (LOH)
  carcinoma in situ, 62–63
  mapping methods, 82

schistosomal bladder cancer, 64
transitional cell carcinoma, 53–56,
    58–61, 82–83
Lymph node, metastasis, 137–138

MCV regimen, bladder cancer response with
    radiotherapy, 152
MDM2, role in TP53 function, 57–58, 87–88
Metalloproteinases
    clonal progression marker, 115
    expression in bladder cancer, 88–89
Mortality, bladder cancer, 5, 11
MVAC regimen, bladder cancer response
    adjuvant radiotherapy, 152
    systemic chemotherapy, 153–155
MVEC regimen, bladder cancer response,
    156
MYC, copy number in cancer, 79–80

N-Acetyltransferase (NAT)
    candidate gene in bladder cancer, 60
    human phenotypes and cancer risk, 8,
        51
NAT. *See N*-Acetyltransferase

Occupational exposure
    aromatic amines, 10
    epidemiology, 11–12
    risk factor overview, 1, 5–6, 11
    screening, 12

Paclitaxel, bladder cancer response, 156
Papillomavirus. *See* Bovine papillomavirus;
    Human papillomavirus
PDEGF. *See* Platelet derived endothelial
    growth factor
Platelet derived endothelial growth factor
    (PDEGF), expression in bladder
    cancer, 90
Prevalence, bladder cancer, 5
Prognosis, bladder cancer, 6, 12, 18–19, 77,
    79, 86, 134, 137–139
PTEN, candidate gene in bladder cancer, 61

Radiotherapy
    chemoradiation, 151–153
    dose, 150
    invasive bladder cancer, 150, 156–157
    postsurgical therapy, 141
    radiosensitizers, 156–157

squamous metaplasia response, 19
RAS, mutation in bladder cancer, 52–53, 63,
    79
RB. *See* Retinoblastoma gene
Reconstruction, bladder, 139–141
Renal cell cancer, viral oncolysis and sponta-
    neous regression, 122–124
Retinoblastoma gene (*RB*)
    alterations in bladder cancer, 58, 84–85
    cell cycle control, 83–84

Schistosomiasis. *See* Bilharzia
SH3BP2, candidate gene in bladder cancer,
    59–60
Smoking
    aromatic amines in cancer development,
        7–8
    cofactor with papillomavirus-associated
        cancers, 36
    dose dependence of bladder cancer
        development, 9
    effects
        bladder cancer severity, 10
        immunotherapy response, 111–112,
            161–162
    risk factor overview, 1, 5–7
    tobacco type and cancer risk, 7
Squamous metaplasia
    bilharzia in promotion, 20–24
    human chorionic gonadotropin expres-
        sion, 19
    prognosis, 18–19
    radiotherapy response, 19
Stage
    effect of age of patient, 13
    effect on survival, 12
    TNM system in staging, 78
Surgery, bladder cancer
    failure, 134–135, 149
    gene therapy, surgical perspective,
        143–144
    histological verification before multi-
        modality therapy, 132–134
    history, 129–132
    imaging, 130, 133
    laboratory models of advanced disease,
        142–143
    multimodal management, 130–131
    neoadjuvant therapy in advanced can-
        cers, 141–143
    pathological factors influencing out-
        come, 137–139

Surgery, bladder cancer (*continued*)
    reconstruction, bladder, 139–141
    superficial tumour control, 135
    transurethral resection of bladder
        tumours, 133, 141, 145

TCC. *See* Transitional cell carcinoma
Telomerase, clonal progression marker, 114
Tobacco smoking. *See* Smoking
TP53
    activation of genes, 85, 87
    angiogenesis inhibition, 90
    apoptosis mediation, 88
    chemotherapy sensitivity effects, 57, 92,
        121, 163
    immunoreactivity and cancer prognosis,
        86
    MDM2 role in function, 57–58, 87–88
TP53
    gene therapy, 110, 120–122
    mutations
        carcinoma in situ, 62–63, 67
        non-bladder tumours, 85–86,
            120–121

    schistosomal bladder cancer, 24,
        63–64
    screening, 68, 86–87, 137
    transitional cell carcinoma, 56–58,
        65, 67, 82, 136–137
Transitional cell carcinoma (TCC)
    carcinoma in situ comparison, 100–101
    chromosome deletions, 53–69, 136
    DNA repair defects, 61
    grading, 78
    loss of heterozygosity, 59–61
    oncogene activation, 52–53
    progression pathways, 50, 65–68
    staging, 78
Transurethral resection of bladder tumours
    (TURBT). *See* Surgery
Tumor necrosis factor alpha (TNFA), cancer
    treatment, 135, 144
TURBT. *See* Transurethral resection of blad-
    der tumours

Vascular endothelial growth factor (VEGF),
    expression in bladder cancer, 90
VEGF. *See* Vascular endothelial growth fac-
    tor

LIST OF PREVIOUS ISSUES

VOLUME 1 1982

No. 1: Inheritance of Susceptibility to
Cancer in Man
Guest Editor: W F Bodmer

No. 2: Maturation and Differentiation in
Leukaemias
Guest Editor: M F Greaves

No. 3: Experimental Approaches to Drug
Targeting
Guest Editors: A J S Davies and
M J Crumpton

No. 4: Cancers Induced by Therapy
Guest Editor: I Penn

VOLUME 2 1983

No. 1: Embryonic & Germ Cell Tumours in
Man and Animals
Guest Editor: R L Gardner

No. 2: Retinoids and Cancer
Guest Editor: M B Sporn

No. 3: Precancer
Guest Editor: J J DeCosse

No. 4: Tumour Promotion and Human
Cancer
Guest Editors: T J Slaga and
R Montesano

VOLUME 3 1984

No. 1: Viruses in Human and Animal Cancers
Guest Editors: J Wyke and R Weiss

No. 2: Gene Regulation in the Expression of
Malignancy
Guest Editor: L Sachs

No. 3: Consistent Chromosomal Aberrations
and Oncogenes in Human Tumours
Guest Editor: J D Rowley

No. 4: Clinical Management of Solid
Tumours in Childhood
Guest Editor: T J McElwain

VOLUME 4 1985

No. 1: Tumour Antigens in Experimental and
Human Systems
Guest Editor: L W Law

No. 2: Recent Advances in the Treatment
and Research in Lymphoma and
Hodgkin's Disease
Guest Editor: R Hoppe

No. 3: Carcinogenesis and DNA Repair
Guest Editor: T Lindahl

No. 4: Growth Factors and Malignancy
Guest Editors: A B Roberts and
M B Sporn

VOLUME 5 1986

No. 1: Drug Resistance
Guest Editors: G Stark and H Calvert

No. 2: Biochemical Mechanisms of Onco-
gene Activity: Proteins Encoded by
Oncogenes
Guest Editors: H E Varmus and
J M Bishop

No. 3: Hormones and Cancer: 90 Years after
Beatson
Guest Editor: R D Bulbrook

No. 4: Experimental, Epidemiological and
Clinical Aspects of Liver Carcino-
genesis
Guest Editor: E Farber

VOLUME 6 1987

No. 1: Naturally Occurring Tumours in Animals as a Model for Human Disease
Guest Editors: D Onions and W Jarrett

No. 2: New Approaches to Tumour
Localization
Guest Editor: K Britton

No. 3: Psychological Aspects of Cancer
Guest Editor: S Greer

No. 4: Diet and Cancer
Guest Editors: C Campbell and L Kinlen

VOLUME 7 1988

No. 1: Pain and Cancer
  Guest Editor: G W Hanks

No. 2: Somatic Cell Genetics and Cancer
  Guest Editor: L M Franks

No. 3: Prospects for Primary and Secondary Prevention of Cervix Cancer
  Guest Editors: G Knox and C Woodman

No. 4: Tumour Progression and Metastasis
  Guest Editor: I Hart

VOLUME 8 1989

No. 1: Colorectal Cancer
  Guest Editor: J Northover

No. 2: Nitrate, Nitrite and Nitroso Compounds in Human Cancer
  Guest Editors: D Forman and D E G Shuker

No. 3: A Critical Assessment of Cancer Chemotherapy
  Guest Editor: A H Calvert

No. 4: Biological Response Modifiers
  Guest Editors: F R Balkwill and W Fiers

VOLUME 9 1990

No. 1: Haemopoietic Growth Factors: Their Role in the Treatment of Cancer
  Guest Editor: M Dexter

No. 2: Germ Cell Tumours of the Testis: A Clinico-Pathological Perspective
  Guest Editors: P Andrews and T Oliver

No. 3: Genetics and Cancer—Part I
  Guest Editors: W Cavenee, B Ponder and E Solomon

No. 4: Genetics and Cancer—Part II
  Guest Editors: W Cavenee, B Ponder and E Solomon

VOLUME 10 1991

Cancer, HIV and AIDS
  Guest Editors: V Beral, H W Jaffe and R A Weiss

VOLUME 11 1991

Prostate Cancer: Cell and Molecular Mechanisms in Diagnosis and Treatment
  Guest Editor: J T Isaacs

VOLUME 12 1992

Tumour Suppressor Genes, the Cell Cycle and Cancer
  Guest Editor: A J Levine

VOLUME 13 1992

A New Look at Tumour Immunology
  Guest Editors: A J McMichael and W F Bodmer

VOLUME 14 1992

Growth Regulation by Nuclear Hormone Receptors
  Guest Editor: M G Parker

VOLUME 15 1992

Oncogenes in the Development of Leukaemia
  Guest Editor: O N Witte

VOLUME 16 1993

The Molecular Pathology of Cancer
  Guest Editors: N R Lemoine and N A Wright

VOLUME 17 1993

Pharmacokinetics and Cancer Chemotherapy
  Guest Editors: P Workman and M A Graham

VOLUME 18 1993

Breast Cancer
  Guest Editors: I S Fentiman and J Taylor-Papadimitriou

VOLUME 19/20 1994

Trends in Cancer Incidence and Mortality
  Guest Editors: R Doll, J F Fraumeni Jr and C S Muir

VOLUME 21 1994

Palliative Medicine: Problem Areas in Pain and Symptom Management
Guest Editor: G W Hanks

VOLUME 22 1995

Molecular Mechanisms of the Immune Response
Guest Editors: W F Bodmer and M J Owen

VOLUME 23 1995

Preventing Prostate Cancer: Screening versus Chemoprevention
Guest Editors: R T D Oliver, A Belldegrun and P F M Wrigley

VOLUME 24 1995

Cell Adhesion and Cancer
Guest Editors: I Hart and N Hogg

VOLUME 25 1995

Genetics and Cancer: A Second Look
Guest Editors: B A J Ponder, W K Cavenee and E Solomon

VOLUME 26 1996

Skin Cancer
Guest Editors: I M Leigh, J A Newton Bishop and M L Kripke

VOLUME 27 1996

Cell Signalling
Guest Editors: P J Parker and T Pawson

VOLUME 28 1996

Genetic Instability in Cancer
Guest Editor: T Lindahl

VOLUME 29 1997

Checkpoint Controls and Cancer
Guest Editor: M B Kastan

VOLUME 30 1997

Lymphoma
Guest Editor: A C Wotherspoon